T0256040

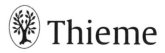

Treating Allergies with F. X. Mayr Therapy

Mobilizing the Body's Self-healing Powers

Harald Stossier, M.D.
Medical Director
Golfhotel Health Center
Wörthersee, Austria

21 Illustrations

Thieme
Stuttgart · New York

Library of Congress Cataloging-in-Publication Data
is available from the publisher

This book is an authorized translation of the German edition published and copyrighted 2001 by Karl F. Haug Verlag, Heidelberg, Germany. Title of the German edition: Allergien erfolgreich behandeln mit der F. X. Mayr-Kur

Translated by Elaine Buchanan, Maria Rain, Austria
Translation edited by Johanna Cummings-Pertl.

© 2003 Georg Thieme Verlag,
Rüdigerstraße 14, D-70469 Stuttgart, Germany
http://www.thieme.de
Thieme New York, 333 Seventh Avenue,
New York, N. Y. 10001, U.S.A.
http://www.thieme.com

Typesetting by Satzpunkt Bayreuth, Bayreuth
Printed in Germany by Gulde Druck, Tübingen

ISBN 3-13-135361-9 (GTV)
ISBN 1-58890-165-3 (TNY)   1 2 3 4 5

Contents

Introduction

Allergies have been increasing for years. We can assume that today, one out of five people have allergies with varying symptoms such as:

- Hay fever in Spring
- Asthma
- Itching skin conditions, rashes or excema
- Joint disorders, and
- Digestive system disorders.

In many cases, a doctor may be able to diagnose an allergy, but much more often, neither the patient nor the doctor considers allergies as the cause of these disorders.

The importance of correctly diagnosing and treating allergies and food intolerances becomes even more obvious when one considers that a link may exist between allergies and alertness, motor activity, sexuality, and food intake. Hyperactivity in children and addiction to certain foods may also be linked to allergies. The same applies to intestinal cramps and cramps of the uterus and other hollow organs. This book provides information for successfully diagnosing and treating allergies and food intolerances.

In recent years, there have been frequent reports of athletes who were able to improve their performance by changing their diets. They achieved these improvements primarily by identifying and omitting foods from their diets that they did not tolerate well. As you read this, you may be thinking that athletes are not like most of us, because they have to achieve peak performance under exceptional conditions of extreme stress.

However, almost everyone can get into stress situations in their daily life that are very similar to those of an athlete competing in an event. We are frequently expected to achieve top performance in our professional and private lives. We even expect such performance from our children and other young people. It should not be surprising that the capacity of our bodies to compensate for such stresses is overtaxed in these situations.

Allopathic medicine has developed precise biochemical concepts for allergies. They clearly define how our metabolism responds, which chemical processes take place, which symptoms are to be expected, and also which therapies are available. Many people, however, do not fit these standard concepts, and their symptoms cannot be explained by them. The following chapters will introduce an expanded concept of allergies, and will illustrate how lifestyle factors can contribute to an increase in allergies.

Allergies are not only a reaction to external substances in genetically predisposed individuals; they also develop as a result of our lifestyle and habits. A major contributor to the development of allergies is the environment, which has changed as a result of our carelessness, and contains many chemical and physically harmful pollutants and irritants. Other contributing factors include our nutritional situation, imbalances in the types of food we eat, and a general lack of healthy eating habits.

This book shows practical ways out of this situation. Change begins in our head, in this case by recognizing our own situation. The next step is to translate this recognition into action. Once we understand our situation, we can more easily overcome challenges to our own health. Changing our way of life can result in decisive improvements for those of us suffering from allergies and its many symptoms. Even if your symptoms do not fit the classic definition of allergies as you know it, we encourage you to read this book. You may be surprised at what you discover about your own health.

What's an Allergy?

The term allergy was coined by the Viennese pediatrician, Dr. Clemens von Pirquet, in 1906. The term originally described the response of the immune system to initial contact with an antigen—a substance that causes an allergic reaction. Pirquet's use of the term included both protective immunity (a beneficial effect) and hypersensitivity or allergic reactions. With increasing knowledge of the biochemical processes involved, the term has come to describe only the hypersensitivity, or over-reaction, of the immune system.

Allergies are part of the adaptation potential of our immune system. They are bound to the same complex processes that our immune system employs to safeguard the integrity of the body. Without our immune system, we would not have suitable defenses against foreign substances of any kind. Let's take the case of a minor infection caused by a virus or bacteria. It necessitates a fast response and intervention by our immune system to prevent damage to our body. Many organs and much of our tissues are involved in this response. Think, for example, of a runny nose, or a swollen throat, as in the case of a cold or flu. Our body's defensive response is subject to numerous biochemical processes. Here is an illustration:

When foreign substance, also called an antigen, enters our body, our immune system responds. It renders the antigen harmless by various means. Which brings us to two important points:

> Antigens are mostly protein structures
> Our immune system has a memory

The second point is significant because, thanks to our immune system, we only suffer certain illnesses once, for example measles and other typical childhood diseases. Our immune system remembers its initial contact with antigen, and can draw on this memory to fight future "invaders" of the same kind. This is the upside of our immune system's memory. The downside is that our immune system's memory of its initial contact with an allergen (a substance that triggers an allergy) can lead to rapid over-reaction every time our body is subsequently exposed to the same allergen.

Patient H.S., male, age 44   *Patient History*

Symptom: a heavy cold for approximately 6 months, sometimes itching skin and a slight rash. Can eat everything, although the patient has the feeling that his condition sometimes worsens after eating.
Various allergy tests showed no indication of an allergy. Cortisone helps considerably, but is rejected as a long term solution by the patient. Six months before onset of the symptoms, he spent a holiday in Italy, which was where his problems started.

Mayr Diagnostics: reveals enlarged abdomen with indication of inflammation in the small intestine, flatulence, and an enlarged liver.
Food Test Results: reveals an intolerance to wheat.

Mayr Therapy: during which, of course, all products containing wheat are omitted. As a result, the patient's cold cleared up completely within 10 days. Regarding the wheat intolerance, a waiting period of 6 months is necessary, during which time various mineral substances will be supplemented.

Our immune system is spread throughout our entire body, which makes sense when we consider that every cell in our body needs to be protected from foreign invasions. This means that the symptoms produced by a immune system response can be very diverse, despite the fact that the bio-chemical processes involved are relatively uniform. These symptoms depend primarily on the location of contact with the allergen in our body, although other factors play a role in determining where the allergy symptoms occur.

The biochemical tools our immune system employs to eliminate foreign substances from our body are essentially those related to inflammation. Blood circulation to the organs or tissues involved is increased, and the region becomes more permeable. This transports more fluids to the area, and recruits enzymes from our white blood cells in an attempt to digest the intruder. This results in a warming or reddening of the area (which can sometimes be visible on the skin surface), and pain may develop.

This normal response of our immune system is also known as normergy (defines a normal process as opposed to the overreaction that results from an allergy).

Stress Response According to Selye

Before we turn our attention to allergic reactions in detail, let's re-emphasize that our immune system's response to stimuli is an essential part of life. Our body needs to be able to correctly identify, process and respond to such stimuli in a series of characteristic phases, and this is a distinctive feature of a healthy body. All body cells can be adequately stimulated. Selye, generally called the "Father of the Stress Field", refers to this series of stages as a stress response.

Each stimulus triggers a brief alarm phase, with a subsequent increased adaptation phase. If our immune system's adaptive capacity is strong, we can appropriately compensate for the stimulus, and normergy (normal sensitivity) is re-established. If, however, the stimulus continues to be present and our response is not adequate, our whole body, or at a minimum, the area that is responding to the stimulus, remains in a state of increased adaptation. This continues until the area involved falls into a state of exhaustion. How long this process takes is important in determining symptoms, but is difficult to establish in retrospect.:.

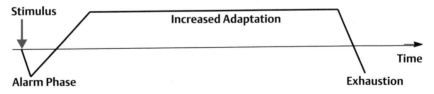

Fig. 1 Selye: Stress Response Phases

According to Selye, if our body remains in the increased adaptation phase for a longer period, this often leads to an allergic reaction. Selye recognized three organ systems that are always involved in a stress response of this kind:

Organ Systems Involved in Stress Response	*Responds to*
● Stomach — Acid–base balance ● Thymus Gland — Immune system ● Adrenal Glands — Hormone system	*Stress*

In this context, an allergy is a stress response of our body. Selye tells us that stress also involves imbalances in our acid-base balance and our hormone systems. The inflammatory response described above always involves, at the same time, a local acidosis (excess acid), and thus confirms Selye's approach. We will discuss hormone balance later in this book; cortisone is one of the hormones involved here that most people are familiar with.

The Austrian physician Dr. Franz Xaver Mayr, in his teachings on the development of illness, described these processes as "normal–excitation–paralysis." Excitation is the immune system's attempt to compensate for, balance, and eliminate the triggering stimulus through increased activity. Paralysis describes the subsequent exhaustion that occurs if the triggering stimulus remains, and the body's own coping mechanism is no longer able to control it.

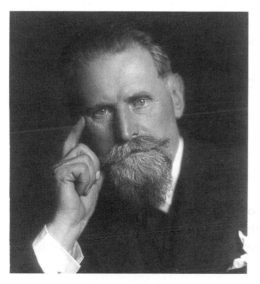

Fig. 2 The teachings of F.X. Mayr were based on his understanding that the digestive system should not be impaired as a result of common nutritional errors. This portrait of the 60 year-old clearly confirms this theory.

Base Substance as Reaction Site for Allergies

The area in our body where the immune system's response to an intruder takes place is called "base substance." This base substance is found throughout our body, in front of the gates to each cell. The base substance is the "reaction site", where the inflammation occurs that fights the triggering agent as a uniform immune system response. As long as the body remains in this response mode, we have a good chance of influencing it. If the process advances, it results in the destruction of cells and organ regions, making therapy more difficult and worsening prognosis. We call this auto-aggression disorder.

The base substance links individual organ structures, and modulates information and metabolism. In this sense, the base substance is also part of a non-specific defense strategy for our body, because it creates milieu factors and influences our body's readiness to react. However, the base substance lacks the ability to remember, which falls to the cellular and humoral components of our immune system. It is also important that a reaction of the base substance in the form of a Selye stress response always precedes a specific immune response (Heine).

If the reaction of the base substance does not proceed correctly, a subsequent immune response will also not proceed properly and may be misdirected. This, in turn, creates the environment for an allergy to develop. This is important because the environmental and nutritional factors we experience as part of our civilized life particularly affect the base substance. Unbalanced nutrition, mineral deficiencies, heavy-metal burdening, inflammation sites, intestinal disorders, and many other factors change the base substance and its behavior. We will come back to this again in the discussion of F.X.Mayr Therapy.

Allergy Characteristics

The over-reaction of our immune system described in the definition above presupposes that a specific stimulus by an antigen leads to a counter-reaction in the form of hypersensitivity. This is not always the case. An antigen can produce a response in one person and have no effect on the next. What makes the difference is the specific reaction of the human body.

Because antigens are molecules (substances) that trigger an immuno-logical response by specific cells of the immune system, we would ex-pect that, strictly speaking, the immune response should be focused on this specific antigen. However, we have found that the immune system can also produce more extensive responses to other substances beyond the triggering antigen. We refer to these as "cross-allergies." Cross-al-lergies can involve many different antigens (see Table 1).

However, even from this overview we can rec-ognize that there are also indirect triggering agents which, strictly speaking, can bring about the same biochemical reactions.

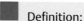 Definition:
An allergy is a response by the im-mune system that far exceeds its original purpose.

Inflammation as Allergy Indicator

Allergies can be triggered by many different factors, but the effects of the allergy on the body are relatively constant. Essentially, they involve excessive inflammatory symptoms with swelling of the tissue involved. This increases the permeability of the base substance, and causes ede-mas (swellings). The effects of such edemas can range from being simply unpleasant to life threatening, depending on the location. For example, an insect sting on the skin leads only to swelling, while a sting inside the throat (which rarely occurs but is possible) can cause the mucous membranes in the respiratory tract to swell, and may impede breath-ing. In extreme cases, this can lead to suffocation through blockage of the respiratory tracts. If the edema involves the mucous membranes in our digestive system, the altered permeability may lead to "leaky gut syndrome," which enables intestinal content to travel into the blood stream. This, in turn, can cause allergies. We refer to this as intestinal autointoxification (see p. 44).

Table 1 Allergy-Triggering Factors

Direct Triggers	Chemical Substances	<ul><li>Food</li><li>Medication</li><li>Environmental pollutants</li><li>Typical allergens: pollen, insect substances</li><li>Household and work place chemicals (Cleaning agents, cosmetics etc.)</li></ul>
	Microorganisms	<ul><li>Bacteria</li><li>Viruses</li><li>Yeast</li><li>Parasites</li><li>Chlamydia</li></ul>
	Foreign Substances	<ul><li>Asbestos</li><li>Plastic</li><li>Dental materials</li><li>Plastics and other synthetic materials</li><li>Heavy metals (amalgam)</li><li>Animal hair, household dust</li></ul>
Indirect Triggers	Transplants	<ul><li>Blood transfusions</li><li>Organ transplants</li></ul>
	Physical Irritants	<ul><li>Temperature</li><li>Radiation–X-rays</li><li>Sun–UV rays</li></ul>
	Metabolism	<ul><li>Acid–base imbalance</li></ul>
	Mechanical Irritants	<ul><li>Pressure</li></ul>
	Psychological Problems	<ul><li>Grief</li><li>Worry</li><li>Fear</li><li>Stress</li></ul>

Other Signs of Allergic Reactions
In addition to swelling, the tissue or organ involved in an allergic reaction starts to heat up and redden. Of course, reddening is only visible if it occurs on the body surface. Overheating and reddening are caused by the release of various mediator substances as part of the biochemical reaction of the allergy. These mediator substances alter the metabolism of the inflamed region. Although they are typical for allergic reactions, they also occur with various other illnesses. Mediator substances are also responsible for any loss of function in the region involved, and for any accompanying pain. In this context, loss of function means the organ or tissue can no longer function normally because of the allergic reaction. With our digestive system, this can result in "leaky gut syndrome". Similar effects can occur in the lungs with asthma, or on the skin with neurodermatitis, for example.

Role of Immunoglobulins
In addition to the relatively non-specific inflammatory responses described above, our immune system can also produce highly specialized defenses—called immunoglobulins. They are divided into several groups: IgA, IgD, IgE, IgG, and IgM.

Immunoglobulins are proteins and include all antibody molecules. They are produced by specialized immuno cells as needed, and display diverse patterns of reaction. Immunoglobulins are antibodies that dock to allergens (or antigens) to render them harmless and enable their elimination. Antigen–antibody complexes of this kind are the triggering agents of unspecific inflammatory reactions, as described previously. Immunoglobulins are also the "memory" of the immune system. Once they have been produced, their level can be increased rapidly when necessary (see Fig. 3).

Besides these specific antibodies, our body also produces a series of enzymes, mediator substances, tissue hormones, and vasoactive amines, which together are important components of any defense response. Their over-production also causes symptoms, and it is primarily vasoactive amines that will interest us in more detail.

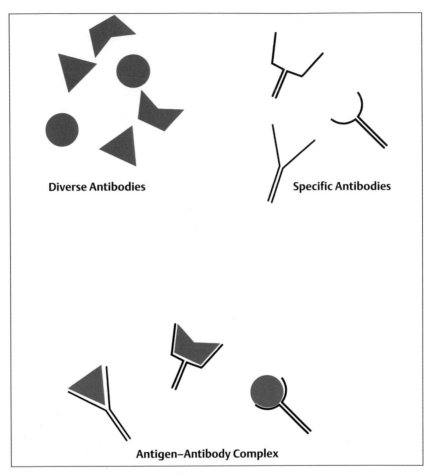

Diverse Antibodies

Specific Antibodies

Antigen–Antibody Complex

Fig. 3 Our immune system responds as follows: Allergens (antigens) find their way into our body (e. g., via skin, lungs, digestive tract). These can be pollen, foods, or other substances. Because they are foreign to the body, the body produces specific antibodies, one for each allergen. These antibodies dock onto the intruding allergen and neutralize it. The resulting antigen–antibody complexes trigger a further defense response, which breaks down these complexes.

Allergy Types

Primary Allergies

Classification of allergies is based on the type of immunoglobin reaction that takes place. In 1968, two researchers, Gell and Coombs, created a division into four different types of reactions, although these constitute only a rough pattern.

Type I—Immediate Hypersensitivity - Anaphylactic Shock

This allergic reaction is mediated by immunoglobin class E. These immunoglobulins constitute only about 0.001 % of all immunoglobulins, but they lead very rapidly, within seconds or minutes, to an immediate reaction. Specific immunoglobulins are produced as a reaction partner of the antigen, causing the release of vasoactive substances such as histamine.

> Warning:
> People suffering from Type I allergies are particularly at risk, as they can suffer anaphylactic shock.

Type I reactions can result in the most acute inflammatory reactions, with anaphylactic shock as the most serious, life-threatening form. Type 1 allergies typically occur with pollen or medication allergies or insect poisoning.

Type II—Early Reaction—Cytotoxic Antibody

Here, allergens are localized on the cell surface. Following initial contact, immunoglobulins of classes M and G are produced (IgG 75 %, IgM 10 % of all immunoglobins). Inflammatory response occurs with a latency period of 12 to 24 hours as a result of cell destruction (cytotoxic reaction). Type II reactions destroy cells because the antibody-antigen combination activates toxic substances. They are found, for example, with blood type incompatibility or rejection of foreign tissue.

Type III—Early Reaction—Immune Complex Hypersensitivity

Here, antigens and the respective antibodies form a complex. This type of reaction occurs when large numbers of antibody-antigen complexes accumulate. It may cause widespread inflammation that damages tissue. Type III allergies typically occur with kidneys and blood vessels disorders. Systemic lupus erythematosus is an example of a Type III reaction.

Type IV—Delayed Reaction or Cell-Mediated Hypersensitivity
This type of reaction occurs when an antigen interacts with antigen-specific lymphocytes that release inflammatory and toxic substances. These attract other white blood cells and trigger a somewhat delayed inflammatory response and tissue injury after approximately 48 to 72 hours. Typically, this reaction occurs with contact eczema and rejection of organ transplants.

The biochemical reactions described so far are involved in primary allergies. They can be triggered by, but are not limited to, foods or food ingredients, for example:

Common *Food* *Allergens*	● Cow's milk ● Chicken eggs ● Various kinds of cereal grains ● Soy and soy products ● Peanut or other nuts ● Fish ● Crustaceans

Other primary allergies can be triggered by insect poison, various chemicals, pollen, foreign tissue, and other direct allergy-triggering agents (see also table 1, p. 16)

Important	Allergic reactions need to be assessed from many different biochemical points of view. Until recently, allergies were classified according to an "all or nothing" system. This is no longer acceptable. Assessment needs to include biochemical findings (as described in the following), improved diagnostics, and therapy that is tailored to the individual. Frequently, several allergic reactions occur simultaneously, or influence each other.

Pseudoallergies

Pseudoallergies do not meet the classification criteria for types I–IV allergies described above, but they present the same or a similar clinical characteristics. People who suffer from pseudoallergies describe a variety of symptoms, which they commonly interpret as food allergies. There are, however, a number of biochemical explanations for these symptoms.

Cross-Allergies

An allergy is commonly defined as a reaction to a specific antigen. If certain components of this antigen happen to be structurally identical to other substances, they will cause the same reaction as these substances. This reaction does not depend on what caused the initial reaction. For example, when somebody who is allergic to cow's milk shows the same reaction when eating beef, we call it cross-allergy.

Cross-allergies can occur even in the absence of contact with the actual allergen. Cross-allergies that are a combination of food allergies and pollen-associated allergies are common. Table 2 lists some frequent combinations.

Cross-allergies need not necessarily occur. They may occur with only one or with several foods, or they may be completely absent. They are difficult to predict and always require a thorough examination of the individual (see Diagnostics).

	Tip
There is hope, even for pollen-associated food allergies. Cooking sometimes helps make a food tolerable. For example, a baked apple is often more easily tolerated than a raw apple. The the same applies to carrots. This solution does not work for histamine intolerance (see p. 23). Histamine is resistant to heat and cold and not impacted by boiling, baking, freezing, or microwaving.	

Table 2 Overview of Cross-Allergies according to Jarisch (●) = potential reaction

	Allergen	Associated Food Intolerance
Pollen	**Pollen**: Hazel–Alder–Birch (March to May)	**Fruit**: - Pome fruit (apples, pears) - Stone fruit (peaches, cherries, apricots, plums) - Kiwis **Nuts**: Almonds, hazelnuts, peanuts, walnuts **Vegetables**: Carrots, celery, peppers, potatoes (raw), etc.
	Grasses Rye (June to July) ----------------------- Mugwort (Artemisia Vulgaris) Ragweed (e.g., Ambrosia aratemisiifolia, Ambrosia trifida) (August)	**Fruit**: Melons (●) **Nuts**: Peanuts (●) **Vegetables:** Eggplant (aubergine) (●), tomatoes -- ------- **Fruit**: Bananas, mangos, melons **Nuts**: Cashew nuts, pistachios **Vegetables/Herbs/Spices:** Anise, basil, caraway seeds, carrots, celery, fennel, marjoram, pepper etc.
	Household Dust Mites	**Seafood**: Crustaceans, clams, mussels, scallops, oysters, **Meat**: Beef (●), pork (●), poultry meat (●)
	Latex	**Fruit**: Avocados, bananas, figs (●), kiwis, peaches **Grains**: Buckwheat **Nuts**: Almonds, sweet chestnuts **Vegetables**: Potatoes (raw)
	Ficus benjamina (and other rubber trees)	**Fruit**: Figs, kiwis (●), pineapples (●), papaya (●)

Histamine Intolerance

Histamine is the most important inflammation mediator substance. It produces a series of biologically important effects in the body. The severity of these effects depends on the level of histamine in the blood.

Table 3 Effects of Histamine (depending on level in blood)

Increase in gastric secretion	1–2 ng/ml
Increase in heart rate	3–5 ng/ml
Drop in blood pressure	6–8 ng/ml
Bronchospasm	7–12 ng/ml
Cardiac arrest	over 100 ng/ml

Histamine is produced by the body and has physiological effects even in minute quantities. Higher levels cause systemic reactions—over-reactions—in the entire body, and may produce typical allergy symptoms. Ten times the normal level of histamine can be life-threatening. Histamine reactions are frequently masked by symptoms that are often attributed to food intolerance, for example:

- Rapid heart beat following meals
- Cardiac arrhythmia
- Shortness of breath
- Asthma symptoms
- Drowsiness, fatigue following meals

Histamine is also a carrier substance in the brain for alertness, motor activity, sexuality, and food intake. Hyperactivity in children and addiction to certain foods can be caused by the effects of histamine. Histamine is involved in the development of pain and leads to contraction of smooth muscles. This can result in intestinal cramps as well as in cramping of the uterus and other hollow organs, which can increase to the point of spasms.

Naturally Occuring Histamine

In the course of allergic reactions, histamine is not only released with type-I reactions, but is contained in all foods, sometimes in very high amounts. Histamine is produced in nature through bacterial decomposition. Histamine is highly effective, and the body must protect itself against excessively high levels. Our first barrier against histamines are our intestines. To break down histamine, the cells of the intestines produce the enzyme diamine oxidase (DOA). This enzyme prevents excessive levels of histamine in the intestines, because this would either lead to local problems or, once the histamine is absorbed, would impact the entire body. Diamine oxidase requires the mineral copper and vitamin B6, which indicates the importance of minerals and vitamins.

Our intestines play another important role in dealing with histamine. Histamine is supplied not only by the food we eat, but by natural bacteria found in the intestines. Our eating habits play a decisive role here. For now, it is important to realize that digestion is always a balancing act between enzymatic digestion and bacterial decomposition. For this balancing act to work, we should supply our digestive system with only the amounts and types of food that it can process completely and in a timely manner. If we overload our digestive system with too much food that our body cannot process efficiently, then this balancing act gets out of control and bacterial decomposition takes over. This results in the development of by-products and end-products of decomposition in our digestive system. For example, high levels of histamine can result from excess intake of protein that is not completely digested, but is instead bacterially decomposed.

Many foods naturally contain varying levels of histamine, and this is discussed below. Digestive health is discussed in more detail in later sections of this book (see pp. 36).

Histamine Content in Foods

Fresh foods contain only negligible amounts of histamine. Histamine is produced by bacteria as food ages. This is especially true for foods in that undergo aging or maturing in the course of their manufacture or preservation, such as the fermentation of sauerkraut, wine, beer, or vinegar, the production of cheese, or the drying of smoked or salted meats. These processes involve microorganisms in the production of aromas. Spoiled meat and fish, of course, contain massive amounts of histamine. Good hygiene and proper handling of food is therefore a prerequisite for low levels of histamine in foods. Histamine levels can show great fluctuations in one and the same group, depending on the type of processing, hygiene, and length of aging process.

> Histamine content increases the longer food is aged or stored.

In addition to foods that contain high histamine levels, there are also foods that release histamine. This presupposes that the histamine is present in the food and is now—similar to a type-I reaction—simply released. This includes citrus fruit, tomatoes, seafood, and above all strawberries. Some food additives may also cause such reactions, for example glutamate, coloring agents, and nitrites.

Table 4 Foods Containing Histamine

- Alcoholic drinks, especially red wine
- Cheese, especially hard cheese, e.g. cheddar, cheshire, gouda, gruyere, swiss
- Chocolate
- Nuts
- Tomatoes
- Salami
- Sauerkraut
- Spinach
- Uncured sausages

Histamine and Medications

Histamine can also be released by various medications, for example, many pain medications such as aspirin. If an allergic reaction to medications is suspected, please consult a doctor about changing the medication.

What Exactly is Histamine Intolerance?

Histamine intolerance is an imbalance between the level of histamine present and the rate the body is able to break it down. Histamine is heat-resistant and cannot be destroyed through heating, boiling, frying, baking, microwaving, or freezing. Allergic reactions to foods depend not only on how much histamine a food contains, but also on our individual threshold and our ability to break down histamine.

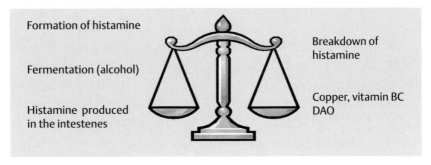

Formation of histamine

Fermentation (alcohol)

Histamine produced in the intestenes

Breakdown of histamine

Copper, vitamin BC DAO

Fig. 4 Histamine Intolerance

Breakdown of Histamine

We have considered the formation of histamine and its effect on the body. Now we will examine the breakdown of histamine more closely. Histamine is a highly active biological substance, and is normally broken down immediately when its level is too high. As discussed in previous sections, this breakdown involves specific enzymes, above all diamine oxidase (DAO). Insufficient breakdown capacity results in an imbalance and in histamine intolerance. The causes for insufficient breakdown capacity can include:

- Congenital enzyme deficiencies
- Side effects of inflammatory gastro-intestinal disorders
- DAO enzyme suppression by various substances, for example medications
- Vitamin and mineral dificiencies
- Overload of breakdown capacity caused by the presence of other substances (so-called biogenic amines) that are broken down by the same enzyme (DAO).

Patient K.D., male, age 43

Symptoms: susceptibility to infection, symptoms of mononucleosis (kissing disease), stomach ache, flatulence, diarrhea, slight gastritis.

Mayr Diagnostics: spastic small intestine, distended abdomen, radix edema, transition between small and large intestine also spastic.
AK Test Results (see p. 58 ff.): generalized hypertonia and histamine intolerance.
Food Test Results: intolerance to cow's milk products and nearly all kinds of cereal grains, parasite infestation, only rice and oats are tolerated.

Mayr Therapy: Following 3 weeks of in-patient treatment on the Mild Clearing Diet and supplementation with orthomolecular substances, symptoms considerably improved. Parasite infestation disappeared; maize, spelt, and millet were tolerated again. Following another 4 weeks of out-patient Mild Clearing Diet and continuation of orthomolecular therapy and parasite therapy, a general state of well-being set in. Cereal grains were tolerated again, only cow's milk products continued to be indigestible. After 1 year, no infection or symptoms whatsoever, repeat of the therapy in a state of general well-being. Abdominal results were clearly improved; AK test indicated normal response, histamine intolerance remained present. Cow's milk products were still not tolerated.

Enzyme Deficiency

Enzyme deficiency is very rarely the cause of histamine intolerance, and has not yet been proven. For the majority of people with histamine intolerance, it does not play a role.

Acute Inflammatory Illnesses

These play a part much more frequently, for example as infections of the intestines. When the acute condition subsides, however, it ceases to play a role.

Chronic Burdening and Illnesses

Illnesses such as colitis or Crohn's disease are often cited in this context, and are important to consider. However, disorders and burdening in the form of an enteropathy according to Mayr (see p. 52) are much more frequently involved. This includes a wide variety of gastro-intestinal disorders, such as chronically inflamed small intestine, fermentation dyspepsia, dysbiosis, yeast or parasite infestations, and putrefaction due to excess consumption of protein. In the long term, all of these conditions overload and exhaust the histamine breakdown system. These disorders tend to be most frequently present in everyday life, but are rarely considered in diagnosing allergic reactions. They will be dealt with in more detail in the chapter on diagnostics and therapy according to F.X. Mayr.

Enzyme Suppression

The enzyme systems that break down histamine also have a built-in feedback loop that prevents them from overshooting the mark. During histamine breakdown, the by-products produced restrict the enzyme systems by sending a signal to the breakdown system that the desired results have been achieved.

Another factor that suppresses the histamine breakdown enzymes is al-cohol, which attacks on two levels: first as a supplier of histamine and second, as a substance that restricts its breakdown. This includes not only alcohol that is ingested, but also the alcohol produced by fermen-tation in the digestive system (enteropathy according to Mayr). In con-junction with dysbiosis (= overgrowth of the intestines with bacteria, yeasts and parasites), the intestines can become the starting point of an enzyme blockade.

Table 5: Examples of Medications that Can Suppress Histamine Breakdown (based on Jarisch, Histamine Intolerance)

Antibiotics	Augmentin
Pain Medications, Analgesics	Metamizole (e.g., Inalgon), Novocain (e.g., Novalgine, Procain)
Cardiac Medications	e.g., Propaphenon, Verapamil (e.g., Isoptine) Rhythmocor, Isoptine
Blood Pressure Medications	e.g., Isoptin
Antidepressants	e.g., Saroten, Typtizol
Cough and Asthma Medications, Expectorants	e.g., NAC (N-acetyl-cysteine) Aeromuc, Mucosolvan

A third important factor for enzyme suppression are medications. Many medications can block the enzyme responsible for histamine breakdown. These range from simple cough medications to antibiotics and cardiac medications.

There are also medications that release histamine—similar to certain foods. This can cause intolerance of a particular medication, or it can trigger or exacerbate any existing histamine intolerance.

> If allergic reactions to medications are suspected, consultation with the prescribing doctor is urgently required to enable the medication to be changed.

Vitamins and Minerals

Enzymes require sufficient vitamins and minerals to break down histamine effectively. Copper is the single most important enabling substance for diamine oxidase (DAO). Copper is also a mineral that is depleted by inflammatory illnesses. For example, chronic inflammatory bowel disorders (enteropathy according to Mayr) can result in serious copper depletion. This, in turn, amplifies the effects of histamine.

Vitamin B6 is also important as a co-factor for the enzyme system. Vitamin B6 deficiency is often found in people with allergy dispositions.

Vitamin C directly influences histamine levels in the blood. The higher the vitamin C level, the lower the histamine. Even with normal levels of vitamin C, histamine levels can be elevated (the increase is extreme in the lower third of the normal range); only upper-normal or slightly raised levels of vitamin C can significantly lower histamine levels. Histamine levels can be lowered immediately with the intake of 1–2 g of vitamin C over several days. At the same time, this improves allergy symptoms, such as rhinitis or asthma.

Orthomolecular treatment, or supplementation of vitamins and minerals, is discussed in more detail on page 112.

Competition for the Histamine Breakdown Enzyme

Histamine belongs to a group of substances called biogenic amines. These substances are produced by the breakdown of protein. The breakdown of protein produces important substances in our body (e. g., adrenaline or melatonin), but also a series of bacterial decomposition products, such as indole, skatole, cadaverine, and thyramine. Some biogenic amines also release histamine, but they are all detoxified by means of the same enzyme system. When several biogenic amines emerge simultaneously with histamine and must be broken down, competition for the enzyme diamine oxidase (DAO) can create a temporary shortfall. The creation of biogenic amines is discussed in more detail in "Digestion and Allergies," p. 36.

Patient History	**Patient D.G., male, age 57**

Symptoms: generalized edemas in the body, 2–3-kg weight gain within a 2-week period, reduced again with diuretics, constantly up and down for years. For 6 to 8 years, reduction in performance, marathon runner despite operations on both hips; foul-smelling, putrid, paste-like stool; palpitations; stomach ache; distended abdomen after consumption of cereal grains.

Mayr Diagnostics: pronounced liver congestion, radix edema, fluid in large intestine, overall fatigue and exhaustion.
AK Test Results: weakness of the liver, positive response to vitamin B3, histamine intolerance, candida (yeast).
Food Test Results: intolerance to cow's milk products, yeast, lactose, potatoes, carrots, and coffee.

Mayr Therapy: A 4-week in-patient Mayr therapy is carried out. After 1 week of strict diet, patient's health is better than it has ever been, good elimination without diuretics, swellings declining, satisfactory weight loss. This is followed by diet of sheep's yogurt and unleavened flat bread, and finally the Mild Clearing Diet. Improvement of all abdominal results. After 4 weeks, the patient can take up sports again, run regularly, feels very well. Of the food intolerances, only intolerance of cow's milk products and coffee remain.

Carbohydrate Intolerance

Until now, we have focused on the link between protein and allergies. However, there are also people who cannot tolerate certain carbohydrates. This does not mean an excess supply of carbohydrate, which would probably lead to fermentation dyspepsia in almost everyone; it refers rather to minute amounts which can produce the same symptoms as allergies.

Fructose Intolerance

The causes of fructose intolerance are similar to those of allergies. Congenital enzyme deficiency is sometimes involved, but is extremely rare. More frequently, the cause of fructose intolerance is an acquired reduction of the bodies ability to absorb sugar molecules in the digestive system. During digestion, carbohydrates are split into individual sugar molecules, which are then actively absorbed by transporters. Fructose intolerance can be caused by a reduction of these transporters.

Of the acquired forms of fructose intolerance, overload and blockage caused by sorbitol is the most prevalent. Sorbitol is an interim product created by the transformation of fructose into glucose. Sorbitol is used to flavor medications and foods, and as a sweetener for diabetics. Simultaneous administration of glucose can stimulate the ability to absorb sorbitol, but also encourages alcoholic fermentation.

Clinical symptoms of fructose intolerance include irritable bowels, flatulence and a tendency toward diarrhea. These symptoms are caused by bacterial fermentation of the fructose that has not been reabsorbed in the large intestine. Symptoms appear about 30 to 45 minutes after the consumption of fructose. Another important consideration is that fructose connects with the amino acid tryptophan in the large intestine and forms nearly insoluble complexes. Tryptophan is transformed into serotonin, which is partly responsible for mood levels and a sense of well-being. Reduced availability of serotonin can cause a reduced sense of well-being, and even depression.

Craving for Sweets

Unfortunately, the symptoms of fructose intolerance are often dismissed as "psychological," due to a lack of knowledge about how to classify or diagnose them. Increased longing for sweets or chocolate cravings are

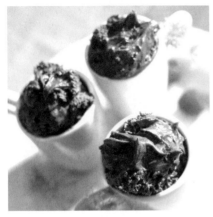

often associated with depression. Understanding the biochemical background of fructose intolerance and its connection with tryptophan and serotonin deficiency helps us understand that when we crave sweets, our metabolism is actually indicating a serotonin deficiency.

Simultaneous intake of glucose along with fructose (or carbohydrates) stimulates any remaining ability to absorb fructose, which releases tryptophan. At the same time, the sugar hormone insulin opens the blood–brain barrier for the absorption of tryptophan. This useful biochemical process gets interrupted by intestinal overload

Fig. 5 There is a clear connection between serotonin deficiency and depression.

conditions. Fructose intolerance occurs very frequently. Also, the breakdown of fructose and tryptophan creates biogenic amines, which, as we saw earlier, are a significant factor in histamine intolerance. This appears to be the reason why histamine intolerance is frequently observed in patients with fructose intolerance.

Patient History	**Patient L.M., female, age 46**

Symptoms: lower back pain, severe muscle tension, recurring helicobacter pylori infection, recurring abdominal complaints, distended abdomen, irritable bowel symptoms.

Mayr Diagnostics: spastic small intestine, flatulence, liver congestion.
AK Test Results: generalized hypertonia with weakness in area of adrenal glands.
Food Test Results: indications of fructose intolerance.

Mayr Therapy: Following 3 weeks of Mayr therapy and avoidance of fructose, practically symptom-free. Continued administration of zinc for hormonal support. No back pain or flatulence whatsoever.

Diagnosing Fructose Intolerance

In addition to paying attention to symptoms and obtaining a precise case history, a hydrogen breath test is often used to diagnose fructose intolerance.

Hydrogen is produced during fermentation of fructose by intestinal bacteria and exhaled via the lungs, which can be measured. If hydrogen level clearly increases following consumption of fructose, this indicates fructose intolerance. Fructose intolerance can also be diagnosed using AK muscle testing, which is discussed in later sections of this book (see p. 62).

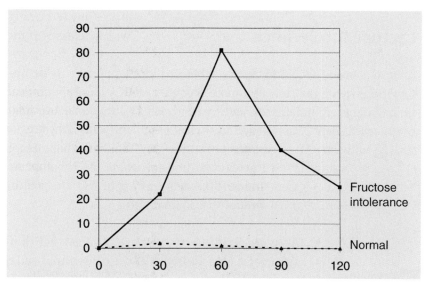

Fig. 6 Hydrogen Breath Test to Diagnose Fructose Intolerance.

Raw fruit and vegetables and foods high in roughage (fiber) almost always cause symptoms. Fructose intolerance is also always associated with zinc deficiency (Ledochowski). Zinc deficiency appears to always go hand in hand with reduced ability to absorb fructose. Zinc deficiencies need to be recognized and treated as a part of the diagnosis and treatment of fructose intolerance.

After the age of 35, folic acid deficiency tends to go along with zinc deficiency. Folic acid is important for the prevention of atherosclerosis (formation of arterial plaque). Folic acid deficiency seems to play a role for some types of cancer.

Table 6 Foods High in Fructose and Sorbitol

- Fruit, fruit compote, preserves, and jams
- Dried fruit
- Fruit juices
- Honey
- Beer

Lactose Intolerance

Lactose is broken down in the digestive system by the enzyme lactase. Genetic enzyme deficiency is more frequent with lactose intolerance than with other intolerances, and seems to follow a marked geographic north–south divide. It is very rare in people of Scandinavian descent (0–3%), while in Africa and Asia, it occurs in 70–100% of the population. In Central Europe and in people of European descent, the enzyme deficiency appears to be present in 10–30% of the population.

As with fructose intolerance, lactose deficiency can also be acquired, and the causes are similar to those of fructose intolerance. 80% of people with lactose intolerance also have fructose intolerance.

The symptoms of lactose intolerance appear about 1 hour after the consumption of food containing lactose, and are caused by bacterial fermentation of lactose in the intestine. This produces irritable bowel symptoms, sometimes cramping, flatulence, diarrhea, and slimy bowel movements.

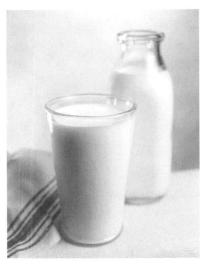

Fig. 7 Milk is a problem for some.

Lactose is found in many foods. Powdered milk or lactose is added, for example, to chocolate, baked goods, processed foods, supplements and medications. Milk contains about 4.5 % lactose.

Fermented milk products (like yogurt or kefir) contain less lactose, because it has to a large extent been fermented by bacteria. There is no difference between cow's, sheep's, or goat's milk in terms of lactose.

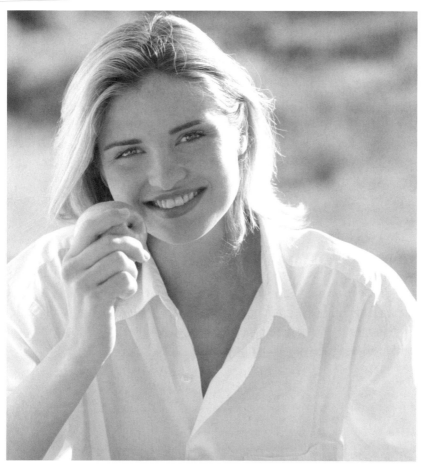

Fig. 8 Easily digestible foods make us healthy and beautiful.

Digestion and Allergies

The task of our digestive system is to process food and create a nutrient solution that can be utilized by our metabolism. Our digestive system begins with the lips and ends with the anus. Nutrition is a process that combines a variety of functions designed to produce a usable nutrient solution.

Feeding ourselves is more than eating; how we process and utilize food is also important. Nutrition is frequently viewed as how much of which foods are eaten. Food quality is an important consideration in these times of food contamination, BSE and environmental pollution. Keeping animals in a manner suitable to their needs, organic farming, and respectful handling of food production are all more important than ever. But we also need to ask ourselves if we can the digest the foods we are about to eat. The Austrian physician Dr. FX Mayr, formulated it very aptly:

"Nutrition is the result of food and individual digestive performance."

We need to be sure that we can metabolize the foods we (want to) eat. Without this important step, healthy nutrition is not possible. Allergies have a lot to do with foreign substances. We define our individuality by means of a specific protein structure that is genetically determined for each individual. There are probably no two people in the world with the same protein structure. Our body also recognizes foreign protein imme-

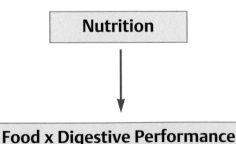

diately, which is very important in the case of blood transfusions and organ transplants. The greatest possible compatibility must prevail between donor and recipient to ensure that an organ is not rejected.

It is the duty of our immune system to recognize compatibility or incompatibility and to react accordingly.

60 % of our immune system is linked to our digestive system. It is here that the decision is made about tolerance or allergy. If the digestive system is working well, allergies rarely occur. Allergies cannot be treated without treating the digestive system.	*Immune System*

We eat foods daily—both of animal and vegetable origin—that contain protein which is foreign to our body. This raises the question as to why we don't reject this foreign protein; on the contrary, we draw nourishment, strength and energy from it.

What makes this possible takes place in our digestive system. Generally speaking, our digestive system is tasked with breaking down individual foods until their "foreign" aspect has been drawn out. With protein, this means that it is broken down into its smallest components, so-called amino acids. These amino acids are then absorbed through the mucous membrane of the digestive system as monopeptides, diopeptides, or tripeptides (separately, in pairs, or in threes). In this form, they no longer possess any component that our immune system would view as foreign. As a result, our body can metabolize these amino acids into protein.

Our digestive system also functions as a barrier. It forms a border between the "inside world" of the rest of our body and the "outside world" of intestinal contents. As long as a particular food is still in the intestines, it is subject to the laws of the digestive process and is not yet intended for the metabolic process. The intestines control what can be absorbed when and where.

With ingested protein, this means that large protein molecules are not absorbed, but first be broken down, as described above. This intact barrier function is an indicator for a healthy digestive system.

As an additional safeguard, all these breakdown and digestion processes are controlled by our immune system. We find this along the entire length of the digestive system—starting with the pharyngeal tonsils, the pharynx, to the lymph nodes of the small and large intestines, and all the way to the appendix. 60–70% of the entire immune system is linked to the digestive system. This makes sense when we consider that large amounts of "foreign material" enter the body daily via the digestive system and must be examined by the immune system for integrity and tolerance.

The part of the immune system that is associated with the intestines constitutes, at the same time, our lymphatic system. Absorbed foods are transported to the liver via the lymphatic fluids, where they are processed further. During this transport, substances are examined. This is another indicator for how meaningfully and wisely nature unites important functions. It also provides a starting point for therapeutic measures.

Digestive Performance

As with everything in the body, digestive function is subject to certain laws. Digestive performance is the most important determining factor. There is no fixed standard for digestive performance, and we can influence it by what, and how and when we eat.
Digestive performance depends on the following factors:
- Constitution
- Fluctuations related to time of day
- Personal behavior

Constitution

Every person is unique in many respects and has been equipped by nature with certain abilities and characteristics. It is more important to learn how to make the most of these assets than to complain that our neighbor has more energy or strength or a better appearance. Everyone can and should use their possibilities constructively and responsibly to retain vitality for as long as possible. We frequently go beyond the limits of our body simply because we want to prove something to somebody, even though this robs more of our reserves than we would like to admit.

We discuss and assess constitution without judging. Normal or abnormal, better or worse are not standards, because everyone has their own constitution. Recognizing our own constitution and acting accordingly is a daily challenge.	*Individuality*

Fluctuations Related to Time of Day

"Eat like an emperor at breakfast, like a common citizen at lunch, and like a beggar in the evening" or "An apple in the morning is gold, at lunchtime it is silver, and in the evening it is lead." These and similar old sayings are still observed by many people, particularly in rural areas.

Many cultures have sayings which express these laws of nature. Chronobiology has been established as a branch of modern medicine that devotes itself to the research of these rhythms. Many or even all metabolic processes are subject to such rhythms: hormone balance, sleep/wake cycles, liver and digestive functions, to mention just a few. Modern research confirms what has been conveyed in the vernacular. Chinese medicine uses an organ clock. It shows us at what time of day an organ system has maximum energy. The organ clock is based on the Chinese meridian interrelations, and shows that digestive performance is at its lowest in the evening.

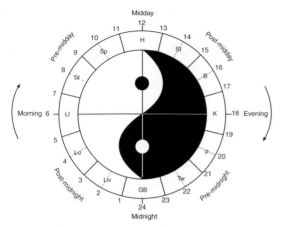

Fig. 9 Living by the Organ Clock:
No raw fruit or vegetables in the evening!

The Organ Clock—A Reflection of our Inner Cycles

If we recognize that digestive performance is at its lowest in the evening, what does this mean for our eating habits? Do we act accordingly? Unfortunately not, most of us do exactly the opposite. Many jobs do not allow for a meal in peace at lunchtime. Some people frown on a mid-day meal because it makes them too tired. Therefore, many people do not eat until the evening, often at a very advanced hour and, on top of everything, much too opulently. Business dinners, social invitations and obligations also take place in the evening, even if it is only to come together in the circle of business partners, friends, or family after a long day's work to find time and peace to eat.

Evenings are the worst possible time for our body and our digestive system to take in and process food. If we observe the rules of the organ clock, our main meal is eaten in the morning and at midday, and only a small, easily digestible meal in the evening, if at all.

It is also advisable not to eat any raw fruit, raw salads, or raw vegetables in the evening. Living, vital food that has not been cooked, or hard to digest foods like whole grain kernels or beans and legumes, place great demands on the digestive system. It is important, therefore, to consciously avoid living according to the frequently heard but misunderstood recommendation: "One can never eat enough raw fruit, vegetables or fiber." This recommendation very frequently results in flatulence, a feeling of pressure, discomfort, insomnia, and many other complaints.

Personal Behavior—What Our Digestive System Needs

Healthy eating habits are vitally important, particularly in the case of allergies! Eating means enjoying, tasting, and getting the most out of food. Eating is more than merely the intake of food. It is helpful to visualize that the digestive system begins with our lips.

Our teeth are tasked with breaking up the food we put into our mouth. Chewing thoroughly is essential for effective digestion, because digestion begins in the mouth. When we chew food

Good digestion starts with thorough, mindful and joyful chewing.

thoroughly, we break up the food and mix it with saliva. This starts the digestive process. Subsequent breakdown and absorption of the food we eat in our digestive system becomes much more efficient when the surface of the food has been appropriately enlarged through adequate chewing. It provides more of a 'target area' for digestive enzymes to work on.

Do you enjoy the taste of the food you eat? Taste can only occur in the mouth. Our mouth is filled with nerve endings that register the quality of the food we chew. By chewing our food well, we produce a saliva-food pulp that the nerve endings in our mouth can then register. The nerve endings then pass this information on to the brain, where it is integrated with our experience and memory as a 'taste sensation'. It is at this point that we "taste" qualities such as sweet, bitter, salty, sour, good-tasting, or "yuck, spit it out." We taste only with our mouth. Once the food we eat leaves our mouth, we no longer taste it, because we can't taste food with our liver, stomach, or small intestine. Thorough chewing heightens our taste experience and adds to the enjoyment of the food we eat. Without thorough chewing, our taste experience is minimal.

In this context, the significance of healthy teeth becomes obvious. Without healthy teeth, proper bite, (and well fitting dentures or other tooth replacements when needed), thorough chewing is difficult, and this first step of our digestive process is impaired.

Chewing also results in stimulation of saliva production. Saliva is important for two reasons. It starts the digestion of carbohydrates in the mouth, and it sends information to our body about the composition of the food we are eating. This information influences the production of digestive juices by the pancreas and small intestine. If we chew our food poorly, salivary production dries up and digestive performance progressively diminishes.

Three Meals a Day?

Besides good chewing and insalivation, it is also important that we give our digestive system sufficient time to digest the food we eat. Frequent snacks between meals disrupt this process more than is generally assumed. Frequent eating is simply not good for us. In general, we can manage very well with two larger meals (morning and midday), and a lighter meal in the evening. The evening meal, if it is needed at all, should be easily digestible, as already mentioned, well chewed, and eaten as early as possible. Our digestive performance is very low in the evening, and observing healthy eating habits becomes particularly important for the evening meal.

The healthy nutrition 'Three Step': Larger portions in the morning and at midday and a smaller portion in the evening—helps to protect us from (digestive) maladies.

Plentiful Clear Liquids

Our metabolic processes require sufficient fluids to work well. We need to supply our body with these fluids by drinking plenty of clear liquids. It is recommended to drink daily approximately 2–3 liters (8 to 12 cups) of:

- good spring water (preferably non carbonated mineral water),
- briefly brewed, light herbal teas, and
- clear vegetable broth

Carbonated beverages like Coca-Cola, Sprite and other soft drinks, energy drinks, fruit juices, vegetable juices, milk, smoothies, alcoholic drinks, black tea or coffee do not count as clear liquids here.

Many disorders of the digestive system such as constipation can be favorably influenced merely by drinking more clear liquids.

The Right Foods

The foods we eat today are frequently very unbalanced, resulting in excess acidity (explained in detail in subsequent sections). Eating the right amount of vegetables and ripe fruit, preferably organic and locally grown, as well as cold-pressed vegetable oils is important.

You Alone Determine How Your Digestive System Reacts
Each of us is individually responsible for our own eating habits. Eating slowly, chewing well, and thoroughly insalivating the food we eat before we swallow is a commitment each of us makes daily at every meal.

Relearning healthy eating habits is one of the most important tasks in Mayr Therapy™. F.X. Mayr described the following cardinal errors of nutrition.

● We eat too quickly (and gulp down our food too hastily). ● We don't chew well (and swallow lumps of food instead of food pulp). ● We don't insalivate enough (and swallow too quickly). ● We eat too frequently (a titbit here, a snack there). ● We eat too much (and keep eating beyond feeling satiated). ● We eat too late in the evening (shortly before going to bed). ● We eat too acidic (too much meat, fish, and cheese). ● We don't drink enough (or incorrectly; only clear liquids count).	*Cardinal Errors of Nutrition According to Mayr*

Therefore, our behavior can influence our digestive performance—in both directions. In a positive sense, through appropriate eating habits and taking advantage of our strengths. In a negative sense, through inappropriate eating habits and overloading our digestion. This overload situation is the first step towards development of disorders.

We should eat only as much as we can break down and metabolize in our digestive system and eliminate via the organs of excretion (intestines, kidneys, lungs, skin). <div align="right">Prof. Pirlet (Frankfurt University)</div>	*Quote*

When parts of the food we eat are not properly digested, they are decomposed by bacteria in our intestines. In this context, "properly" means timely and completely. Proper digestion is always a balancing act between enzymatic digestive performance and bacterial decomposition.

Normally, enzymatic digestion will leave just enough for intestinal bacteria to thrive in a symbiosis (mutually beneficial coexistence), but not take over control. However, if we overload our digestive capacity by neglecting healthy eating habits, our intestinal bacteria receive so much food that misdigestion occurs. Depending on the type of food, misdigestion means either fermentation (from carbohydrates) or putrefaction (from protein). Both seriously disrupt the integrity of our digestive system and pave the way for allergies.

Link between Intestinal Autointoxification and Allergic Reactions

Overloading our digestive capacity leads to misdigestion. For example, any excess protein we eat is bacterially decomposed instead of enzymatically broken down. The average diet today contains too much protein, often double or even triple the daily requirement.

Decomposition of this protein by bacteria, also called putrefaction, produces biogenic amines. We have already met one of the main representatives of biogenic amines—histamine—as the most important trigger of allergic reactions. But bacterial decomposition in our digestive system also produces other biogenic amines: cadaverine, putrescine, spermine, spermidine, thyramine, indole, and skatole. Some of these, such as spermidine, release histamine themselves; others intensify the effect of histamine, because they are broken down by the same enzyme (see p. 30).

Excess carbohydrates in our diet are subject to fermentation in our intestines. In this case, the effect on allergies is more indirect. Fermentation produces alcohol, acids, and gas. Both alcohol and acids impair the function of the digestive system, especially its barrier function. Alcohol dissolves fat, which can cause the mucous membrane of our digestive system to develop leaks or holes, figuratively speaking. This condition is also referred to as 'leaky gut syndrome'. The intestines become permeable for substances from within the digestive system that should not be absorbed, or at least not yet. This allows incompletely digested fragments of protein to make their way into the body. The intestine-associated immune system recognizes this fragment as foreign protein and, following sensitization, reacts allergically.

This process is called autointoxification or self-poisoning from the intestines.

We have also met alcohol as an inhibiting factor for breakdown of histamine. Fermentation due to excessive consumption of carbohydrates reinforces allergy symptoms. The most unfavorable situation is misdigestion that combines both fermentation and putrefaction.

Summary

Misdigestion processes such as fermentation and putrefaction disrupt the integrity and function of our digestive system on several levels:
- Misdigestion compromises the barrier function of the digestive system. Leaks appear in the intestines and make them permeable for intestinal contents (leaky gut syndrom).
- Food is not properly and completely digested. This produces biologically highly effective substances, which can trigger allergies.
- Loss of the barrier function enables toxins to be partially absorbed into the body, a process described as autointoxification.
- Both fermentation and putrefaction and the immune system's response to the resulting toxins use up minerals in order to neutralize the situation.
- Treatment of fermentation and putrefaction, as well as long-term avoidance of the same, can prevent many allergic reactions.

Dysbiosis, Candidiasis, Parasites

An inconceivably large number of bacteria live in our digestive systems. It is assumed that the number of bacteria is larger than the number of cells in our body. These bacteria live in symbiosis, which means that they have certain tasks in the digestive process. An imbalance of the normal healthy intestinal flora (which means all bacteria that live in our intestines) is referred to as dysbiosis. Dysbiosis can have many causes: some illnesses, antibiotic therapy, or, as already explained, bad dietary habits. Burdening as a result of amalgam—of which the main representative, mercury, has the effect of an antibiotic—likewise leads to dysbiosis.

Dysbiosis can only effect the relationship of individual bacteria to each other. Individual strains are diminished, others increased. An increased presence of bacteria that lead to putrefaction, such as *proteus, pseudomonas,* or *clostridium,* produces a series of biogenic amines from the breakdown of protein. These biogenic amines play a decisive role in histamine intolerance.

Candidiasis

Dysbiosis can also indicate the presence of yeasts in the intestines, the main representative of which is *Candida albicans.* Although there are still varying opinions as to the role of yeasts as a cause of illness, candidiasis clearly paves the way for allergies and/or intolerances. Candidiasis meets all the criteria for intestinal disorders that lead to allergies:

- *Candida albicans* has the ability to release histamine.
- *Candida albicans* produces a series of toxins, of which about 60 have been identified in more detail.
- Fermentation alcohol (produced by candida) blocks the breakdown of histamine.

Together, the toxins released by candida cause disintegration of the mucous membrane of the digestive system and thus, disruption of the bar-

Table 7 Examination for Candidiasis and Food Intolerances

Total number of examinations	148
Number of people with candidiasis	76
Number of people with food intolerance	74
Baker's yeast	61
Cow's milk products	50
Wheat	29

rier function. Once again, we have the "leaky gut syndrome", which creates an environment for autointoxification, as previously described. Our observations show that candidiasis is present in at least 50% of patients. More than 90% of these cases also involve intolerance to one or more foods. Candidiasis is a 'red carpet' for food intolerance.

- Multiple food intolerances are the rule; in only two cases of candidiasis was there no food intolerance.
- The process can also be reversed—a food intolerance can lead in the long term to dysbiosis or candidiasis.

Parasites

Parasites cause similar problems as yeasts. Parasites are scroungers that live mainly in the digestive system at the expense of their host - our body. Among these are a wide variety of worms, rickettsias, amoebas, and *Lamblia intestinalis*. Increased travelling abroad has made many formerly "exotic" parasites more common than one would expect. Parasite infestation is often associated only with lack of hygiene, which is not correct. We have to assume that parasites occur more frequently than is generally assumed; estimates indicate in up to 25% of the western population.

Symptoms of Parasite Infestation
Clinical symptoms of parasite infestation, or parasitosis, are gastro-intestinal disorders, itching on the body, especially around the anus, and poor general health with tiredness and exhaustion. These often completely recede into the background or are regularly observed as recurring at intervals of varying length, interspersed with symptom-free periods. In children, anaemia and developmental disorders can be caused by worm infestation and should also always be taken into consideration. However, parasite infestations frequently exist without the classic symptoms.

Patient History	**Patient: S.M., male, age 13**
	Symptoms: feels well in general, however diminished school performance, decreasing concentration, is active, does sports, but is lacking in strength.
	Mayr Diagnostics: firm abdomen, enlarged liver, sounds of liquid (squelching) in lower right abdomen. *AK Test Results:* normotonic (normal) muscle reaction, weakness in the area of small intestine which is balanced by means of the parasite medication pantelmine. This indicates parasite infestation. Several mineral deficiencies.
	Mayr Therapy: During check-up 3 weeks later, patient reports short-term improvement with subsequent deterioration. Repeated cycle of therapy twice more, then continuing improvement. After 2 months, condition stabilizes, physical performance increases. Good concentration, improving school performance.

As soon as a parasite is recognized as foreign by the body, special defense cells, so-called eosinophil granulocytes, attempt to eliminate it. Increased eosinophilia (group of white blood cells) should be an indicator to consider parasitosis. However, normal levels of eosinophilia does not rule out parasitosis.

Link between Parasites and Allergies

Parasites cause allergic reactions in a wide variety of ways. They are a foreign protein which can cause allergic reactions. The activity of eosinophil leucocytes releases histamine. Parasites produce a series of metabolic substances. All these factors produce a micro-milieu in our body which creates a supportive environment for the parasite, but is directed against the host—us. In this milieu, we find biogenic amines as the products of putrefaction, but also a whole range of fermentation alcohols. The latter are sometimes specific to individual parasites.

Summary	Dysbiosis, candidiasis, and parasitosis produce similar effects. Dysbiosis, irrespective of cause and type, leads to a change in the digestive system milieu. This encourages allergic reactions and leads to intestinal autointoxification by disrupting (or destroying) the integrity of the digestive system. The goal of treatment is therefore restoration of a healthy digestive system.

Lymph System and Allergies

The lymph system is part of the body's defense strategy. The term lymph means water. In this case it refers to the fluid that flows in tissue crevices. Lymph fluid collects in very delicate lymph channels, similar to those of the blood's circulatory system, which run through the entire body as a transport system. Situated in these lymph channels are the lymph nodes. They filter the lymph fluid and, in coordination with the immune system, examine it for antigens. The lymph nodes contain immune-competent cells (lymphocytes) that can immediately act immunologically if necessary. These defense centers are found in areas where potential foreign matter is expected; throughout the entire digestive system, beginning in the throat, the tonsils, the so-called Payer's glands, and the appendix. 60 to 70% of the immune system is connected to the intestines.

Similar conditions exist in the lungs, where foreign substances are taken in via inhalation of air. Our thymus gland, spleen, and bone marrow also belong to the immune system in a closer sense. They carry out the immune system's memory function; which means that they produce special cells that react upon second contact with an allergen.

How the Lymph System Works

In the gastrointestinal tract, reabsorption of food takes place via the lymph system. The lymph system can also be compared to a sewer system. It carries waste products away and delivers them to the sewage plant—the lymph nodes. After cleansing has taken place, the now clean water is redirected into the circulatory system. The lymph nodes are responsible for cleansing, detoxifying, and recognizing anything foreign, and for passing this information on to the entire body.

As with everything else, the lymph system can be overloaded. If the quantity of harmful substances and thus the necessity for cleansing is greater than the capacity to eliminate the intruder at the time, it leads to an expansion of the sewage plant—the lymph nodes become enlarged. If the quantity of disruptive substances persists, the transport system becomes congested.

The radiologist Weiss described this congestion of intestinal lymph as "radix edema," because lymph congestion (edema) becomes both visible and perceptible in the area of the suspension system of the small intestine (the root = radix). As a radiologist, he was able to prove this through X-ray imaging. In Mayr diagnostics, it is palpable as a sometimes very hard resistance deep in the abdomen.

From the *Practice*	A colleague who was carrying out a Mayr therapy also examined his wife. Having felt "something hard" in her abdomen, he phoned in a very distressed state. As an intensive-care doctor, he had seen such findings only in cases of advanced cancer. With Mayr diagnostics, we were able to reassure him. The result clearly showed a radix edema, which we confirmed with further examinations.

Effects of Radix Edema

The more pronounced this edema is, the more frequently it causes a shifting of the loops of the small intestine, together with irritation and pain in the spinal column and congesting the entire lymph drainage—both from the upper body and from the legs. Swelling in the legs, but also in the chest (particular attention must be paid in the case of women!) always arouse suspicion of a congestion of the radix.

If inflammatory processes also set in, it can cause "pain of unidentified origin," sometimes affecting the abdomen but more frequently the spinal column. This is the root cause of many back problems of "unclear" origin.

We must assume that all cases of digestive disorders in the form of fermentation and putrefaction involve not only a disruption of the intestinal barrier function. The substances which are able to enter the body because of this disorder also force the intestine-associated immune system to respond. This results in congestion of the intestine-associated immune system, and effects the entire body.

Other organ systems also receive the "allergy information" and react accordingly. Finally, the toxins that have found their way into the body have to be detoxified and rendered harmless. This takes place, for example, in the liver.

Both classic manual lymph drainage and manual abdominal treatment carried out by a Mayr doctor are important therapeutic measures in the treatment of lymph congestion. In addition, there is a range of good, effective medications available that likewise improve lymph circulation. Care must always be taken that an adequate amount of liquid is drunk, as without liquid it is impossible for the lymph to flow.

A great deal of patience is necessary in the therapy of lymph congestion, since the lymph system only regenerates itself slowly. However, freedom of symptoms, or at least a reduction of the same, can be achieved quickly when therapeutic guidelines according to Mayr are observed.

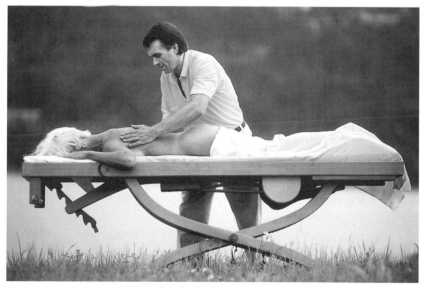

Fig. 10 Lymph drainage detoxifies the body.

F.X. Mayr Diagnostics

The Austrian physician Dr. Franz Xaver Mayr developed his system of diagnostics and therapy at the beginning of the last century. This could be considered 'ancient' in present-day medicine, but Mayr's findings are as current and relevant today as they were a 100 years ago.

While in medical school, Mayr started asking questions about what makes a healthy digestive system; logical questions to which he received inadequate answers, both as a student of medicine and later as a practicing doctor.

Three Essential Questions	1. How can health be recognized? 2. Where does health end and disease begin? 3. What characterizes a healthy digestive system specifically and a healthy person in general?

As a result, Mayr dedicated his medical activities to these questions and began researching the digestive system. Mayr treated all of his patients as if their digestive systems were out of order, irrespective of whether they complained of such disorders. He justified this with lack or deficency of knowledge of the above-mentioned criteria of a healthy digestive system, and made his patients fast in a wide variety of ways. At the same time, he cleansed their digestive system and paid attention to healthy eating habits. The results of this regime were at first completely unexpected, and later specifically predictable.

By improving the digestive system not only did specific digestive complaints disappear, but also complaints which, at least at first glance, had absolutely nothing to do with digestion—namely heart–circulatory disorders, lung or kidney disorders, and many more.

Improvements in health always follow certain rules and can be pursued until a state of ideal health is achieved.

Even those who consider their digestive system healthy display deviations from a state of ideal health and are thus to be considered as burdened or clogged.

Recognizing these rules, Mayr developed a picture of an "ideally healthy person." As with a puzzle, he fitted together all diagnostic characteristics of ideally healthy organs he found to form a picture, an idea. Mayr himself recognized and emphasized that he never found all signs of ideal health at the same time in one person. May developed something completely new in the field of medicine—a coherent and defined ideal picture of a healthy person, as opposed to normal medical findings and values.

Diagnostics of Health

Mayr diagnostics can determine how and to what extent an individual deviates from this ideal at any moment. Latent disorders can be determined before they manifest as disease. Burdening can be objectively evaluated even before standard laboratory test results, ultrasound scans, or other modern procedures indicate deviations. During treatment, Mayr diagnostics can determine whether the path taken leads to improvements; that is, in the direction of the ideal state or not.

Mayr, therefore, developed diagnostics of health. How refreshing this is, when medicine is usually concerned with sickness. And if health is not only the absence of illness, but an independent strength within us, then we must not only maintain health, but also promote it. Vitality and enjoyment of life are therefore the aim of the recuperation process.

Ideal health is a state which requires no further improvement. All organ systems perform optimally with a maximum of effectiveness and a minimum of effort. This economy characterizes Mayr's concept of health. To function economically, our tissue and organs must meet certain optimal conditions regarding shape, size, position and tonus. These conditions of optimal shape and function are characteristics of Mayr diagnostics.

Mayr diagnostics primarily employ our five senses. This does not mean abandoning modern methods of diagnosis, but rather preceeding these with simply looking, perceiving, manually examining, determining the quality of living systems, interpreting these and then acting accordingly.

Mayr, of course, did not limit himself merely to the digestive system, but described signs of health for the entire body. An appropriately trained Mayr doctor will therefore examine all of these criteria at the beginning, before making a diagnosis. It would be beyond the scope of our topic to portray all examination procedures here, so this book will focus on a few of the details that are important with allergies.

Role of the Abdomen in Mayr Diagnostics

A healthy abdomen can be defined by its shape and size. Mayr described several possibilities of measuring size. (Measurements according to Mayr are always given in so-called "finger-widths"; the use of measuring tapes is possible but not absolutely necessary.) Figure 11 shows that the size of a healthy abdomen corresponds approximately to the span of an outstretched hand.

Deviations in size occur when individual organs of the digestive system require more space. This causes not only abdomen to increase in size, but also a change in the boundaries of individual organs, where needed.

In addition to size, the state of tension—tonus—is also a criteria for assessment. An ideally healthy abdomen is soft, elastic, and can be examined well and painlessly. Individual organs can change their position for a short time, but return quickly to their normal positions. Theoretically, the abdomen can be probed to such an extent that the spinal column can be felt on its rear wall. This tonus keeps the organs in their place and is partly responsible for their optimal functioning.

It is precisely this tension or tonus that alters in the case of allergies. At the beginning of the book, it was mentioned that an allergy constitutes an over-reaction. Selye speaks of an initial alarm phase and later an increased adaptation phase. Mayr calls this phase "excitation." It describes increased tissue tonus, a state of irritation. Since the digestive system possesses a large proportion of muscle, this will determine the symptoms. The abdomen becomes firm, partly hard. It can also react spastically, or by cramping from time to time. This occurs initially following the ingestion of the allergen; later, when the irritation occurs more frequently, the abdomen remains in this state of tension almost constantly. The symptoms can range from colicky pain to spastic constipation.

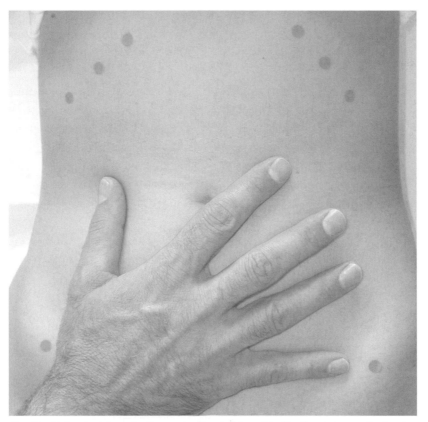

Fig. 11 Abdominal Examination according to Mayr. Ideally, the abdomen is about as big as the hand. Thumb and forefinger of the examining hand should touch the arch of the ribs (dotted line). The abdomen in this picture is enlarged: there is space between the fingers and the arch of the ribs. It no longer meets ideal conditions.

Another diagnostic criteria is the ability of individual organs to move and shift, both together and in relation to each other. With allergies, the inflammation triggered by the mediator substances can reduce or even eliminate this mobility. This eliminates change in pressure as a motor for peristaltic, blood, and lymph drainage, and encourages congestion. Congestion of the radix, the small intestine, has already been described (see pp. 50).

In connection with the inflammatory response, this lack of mobility can manifest itself in passing on the pulsations of the abdominal aorta (large abdominal artery) to the abdominal wall. Therefore, a perceivable, or even visible pulsating spot on the abdominal wall indicates irritation of the abdominal lymph. It can be assumed to indicate congestion and thus immunological burdening.

An existing dysbiosis is characterized by fermentation and/or putrefaction. Fermentation produces alcohol, acids, and gas. This formation of gas leads to a distended abdomen, in serious cases to an extremely tense drum-belly. Many patients also report feeling bloated after every meal (or after certain foods = indication of food intolerance). With some people, this is so extreme that they have to undo their belts after a meal (but not because of the quantity consumed!).

Although gas also results from putrefaction, it is not as pronounced. But the sulphur compounds of putrefaction often emanate foul smells.

These varying indications of burdening of the digestive system occur alongside each other and simultaneously. Changes in tonus and elasticity lead to changes in position of the individual organs. As a consequence, the functioning of the entire digestive system is impacted.

These processes follow characteristic laws and are known as enteropathy according to Mayr, which defines tendencies to develop illness resulting from the digestive system. We can assume that in the course of this enteropathy, misdigestion produces toxic substances, which are then absorbed and distributed throughout the body. This intestinal autointoxification leads to a range of so-called "remote symptoms". These were summarized by Mayr as humoral-diagnostic indications. Examples include skin color and texture, distended blood vessels in the skin (known as spider veins or couperose), and the condition of nails, skin, or eyes.

Table 8 Mayr Diagnostics Details in the case of Allergies

- Inflammatory fecal belly
- Radix edema
- Spastic intestinal sections
- Dysbiosis
- Autointoxification from the intestines

Recognizing Allergies/Intolerance

It is known today that allergies are the cause of many illnesses. Among these are neurodermatitis, bronchial asthma, various contact eczemas, hay fever, and irritable bowel symptoms. A type-I allergic reaction of the immediate type with genetic disposition is referred to as atopy. There is also a range of complaints and symptoms which, although they point to an allergy or intolerance, do not fit into the classic allergy pattern. Among these are headaches, migraine, chronic sinusitis, cardiac arrhythmia, stomach complaints, gastrointestinal disorders, irritable bowels, skin diseases, and many more. One should also not be put off by "modern" diagnosis such as fibromyalgia syndrome or polymyalgia rheumatica.

Patient History

> **Patient F.D., male, age 23**
>
> *Symptoms:* irregular abdominal complaints for approximately 1 year, sometimes diarrhea, then normal stool again. Blood in stool once. Frequent abdominal cramps, loss of weight, symptoms usually, but not only after meals, more unpleasant at night. Many examinations failed to give a clear indication, possibly Crohn's or colitis. Intensive questioning revealed an enormous burden of stress as the cause.
>
> *Mayr Diagnostics:* showed pronounced spasticity of intestines, partially filled with gas, enormous sensitivity to pressure, and lymph congestion. Further examinations indicated histamine intolerance with intolerance to all kinds of cereal grains.
>
> *Mayr Therapy:* After 4 weeks of in-patient Mayr treatment, with avoidance of the nontolerated foods, gradual improvement, readiness to talk about the cause.

With diagnosis such as "unclear genesis" and "psychosomatic," allergies or intolerance should always be considered. The extensive field of gynecological disorders, from menstrual problems to menopausal complaints, can involve allergies. In the area of exercise or athletics, constantly recurring complaints of the musculoskeletal system, especially of the muscle and tendon bases, can indicate an intolerance or allergy.

> Disorders that occur in connection with the consumption of specific foods or as a result of specific external influences, e. g. in the sleeping/living area, usually involve allergies or intolerance.

Classic Allergy Diagnostics

Classic allergy diagnostics encompasses a thorough case history and assessment of existing medical results as well as a series of examinations and laboratory tests, some of which will now be briefly described.

Laboratory Tests

In the laboratory, numerous parameters can be tested. Determination of the individual immunoglobulin is standard. Above all, the increase in immunoglobulins E indicates a type-I immediate reaction. A parasite infestation also shows high levels of immunoglobulin E. Testing for allergen-specific IgE antibodies is more precise than testing for immunoglobulin.

In recent years, so-called "immunotests" have established themselves in the field of food testing, whereby the reactions to immunoglobulin class G are examined in the test-tube. This would most likely correspond to a type-III reaction according to Gell and Cooms.

Provocation Tests

More frequently, provocation tests are carried out on the skin to prove a type-I reaction. For this, certain allergens are applied to the skin or inserted into the surface of the skin by means of various procedures. The reaction of the skin is then observed after approximately 20 minutes (immediate type), and again after 24 hours for possible late reactions. There are standardized allergy mixtures available for these tests.

To prove contact allergies (late type IV reaction), the allergens in question are usually applied to the skin of the back. Reactions occur, as expected, after 2 or 3 days, or even later.

Provocation with allergens can also be carried out on the eye or as an inhalation provocation via the nose. Both tests are easy to carry out; however, they can also be unpleasant because corresponding clinical reactions are judged to be proof of an allergy. All provocation tests could lead to acute reactions in the form of an anaphylaxis. For this reason, precautionary measures in case of an emergency must be taken.

In addition to test procedures to verify the allergies of types I–IV, there are some procedures which, although they are much too involved for routine diagnostics, have proved themselves very useful for specific questions.

Lymphocyte Transformation Test

This is a special test to determine the immunological status of lymphocytes with regard to specific antigens. In this way, a differentiation of the immunological response to questionable allergens can be carried out. The effort required and the costs are relatively high so that only specific questions, e. g., an intolerance to dental materials, justify application of this test.

Histamine Release Test

This test measures the release of histamine from lymphocytes through an allergen. The test does not always show the same results as other tests, it is costly and not simple to implement. This test is also not appropriate for routine diagnostics.

Extensive Allergy Diagnostics

With due respect for the various tests, it is nevertheless recognized that they do not always produce breakthroughs in allergy diagnostics. On the contrary, experts agree that a precise case history and exact questioning form the basis of diagnosis and that the tests constitute only an additional, albeit important, tool.

Comprehensive diagnostics require a holistic approach, which would include

- F.X. Mayr Diagnostics
- Diagnostics using applied kinesiology (AK)
- additional special laboratory tests

F.X. Mayr Diagnostics

You have already met the principles of Mayr diagnostics (see p. 52). The criteria for allergy disposition and intolerance are

- Enteropathy according to F.X. Mayr
- Inflammatory fecal belly
- Spastic intestine sections
- Radix edema
- Signs of a dysbiosis
- Signs of intestinal autointoxification with remote symptoms

Mayr diagnostics can be used to diagnose allergy symptoms, but cannot differentiate between individual allergens. The abdominal results for food intolerance are comparable to those of pollen-associated allergy or histamine or fructose intolerance. These requires further differentiation, for which applied kinesiology has proven valuable. Mayr diagnostics are, however, important for checking progress and for assessing positive and negative reactions during therapy. They provide information about the current state at any given time.

Applied Kinesiology

Applied kinesiology, hereafter referred to as AK, originates from the U.S., and was developed by George Goodheart, DC, a chiropractor. Coming from the manual medical field, he soon recognized the interrelation of structural problems and internal organs, their metabolism and nutrients in the form of minerals, vitamins, and trace elements. Of course, the emotional side is also integrated, giving us the so-called "triad of health" as a comprehensive working hypothesis.

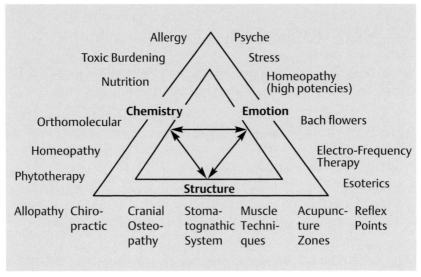

Fig. 12 Triad of Health

Muscle testing is used as a diagnostic criterion. What is decisive is the response of the system to previously set and clearly defined irritations, rendered visible and perceptible through the muscle test.

Definition	AK is primarily a diagnostic method; with its help, the reaction situation of living biological systems can be examined quickly and simply.

Muscle Testing as a Central Source of Information

Properly implemented muscle testing is prerequisite for attaining reliable results through AK. It requires having a defined test position for each muscle, corresponding to the course and function of that muscle.

The patient is asked to contract the muscle to be tested with maximum strength against the resistance of the examiner. The examiner exerts a counter-pressure long enough to perceive that the patient has reached his/her individual level of strength.

The examiner then increases the pressure by a maximum of 5% and checks whether the patient withstands this increase in strength. Ideally, this examination pressure is tolerated without any problem, which indicates "intact neuromuscular integration."

It is important that the muscle test is seen as neither a contest nor an opportunity for the examiner to try to prove his/her superior strength. It is far more a matter of perceiving the patient's level of strength and of selecting the test pressure and duration in such a way as to attain exact and reproducible results. Each muscle test lasts no longer than 3 to 4 seconds. This tests not only the muscle, but also the patient's regulatory response and stress adaptation. The result of the muscle test provides us with information on how the patient reacts to irritations that are clearly defined by us, for example an allergen.

Possible Results of Muscle Testing

Biologically Correct Muscle Response— Normotonic Muscle Test Result
If a muscle reacts strongly when the test is carried out properly, it indicates that the system being tested tolerates slight additional stress. However, the muscle can be temporarily weakened by a normal level of weakening irritations. Normotonic muscle test results signify a balanced, presently stable system which recognizes both positive and negative irritations and is capable of reacting to them.

The Weak Muscle

A muscle response is referred to as weak when the patient can no longer adequately counteract the additional test pressure in the muscle test described above.

The Constantly Strong Muscle—Hypertonic Muscle Response

Here, the muscle remains strong at all times during the test. It does not respond to normally weakening measures, but remains constantly, and therefore inappropriately, strong.

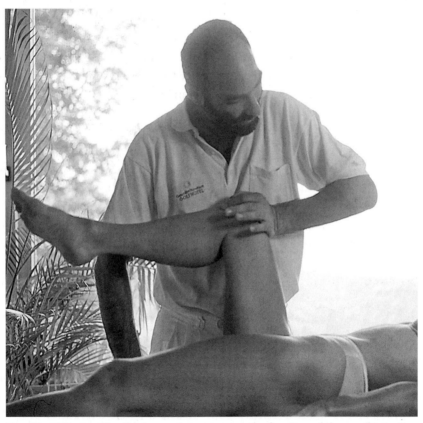

Fig. 13 AK test on the thigh muscle to examine the function of the small intestine meridian in the case of an allergy.

Significance of "Normotonic," "Hypertonic," and "Weak" Muscle Response for Allergies

These three possible muscle responses correspond essentially to the phases of stress response according to Selye. With AK muscle testing, we therefore examine the state of stress as well as a patient's individual adaptation and response. In accordance with Selye's comprehensive definition of stress, we can and must examine all of these factors with AK, because we want to guide the patient back to a normal response state. With AK, we can find out what is beneficial for the individual, and what can be helpful in enabling a return to a normal response state. AK can also determine burdens due to foods or other allergens.

Initially, it is difficult to imagine that such a simple examination can be relied upon for our investigation into allergies or intolerances. It was Goodheart's intention to provide the medically trained specialist with an additional source of information for diagnosis. However, since muscle testing is relatively simple to learn and is not invasive, many medical lay people have begun to use it. It has also been partially modified, expanded, or renewed. Every change to the original course of the procedure has damaged the method more than helped it. Today, "kinesiology," as well as various variations of it such as psycho kinesiology, edu-kinesthetics, and physioenergetics, are carried out by medical lay people. Kinesiology is sold to patients as a natural-healing/holistic method of diagnosis, as the basis for social counselling and psychosomatic treatment, or as an energetic holistic method. Despite the dubious practice of the respective "kinesiologists," they are frequently amazingly successful.

> Stress is the sum total of all adaptation processes and responses of body and mind with which a living being reacts to its environment and to internal and external demands.
>
> Selye

Lay kinesiologists, however, frequently lack the specialized qualifications required to investigate allergies and/or intolerances. Often, too much importance is attached to one side of the "triad of health," namely the emotional side, resulting in a distortion of the results.

Even if "kinesiology" does not directly cause damage, I am repeatedly confronted with statements such as "I have already been to a kinesiologist,

Patient History	**Patient H.S., female, age 40**
	Symptoms: gastro-intestinal disorders since childhood, mostly constipation. Taking various laxatives. Various diets, finally consultation with a social counselor. AK testing by social counselor revealed conflicts in earliest childhood. The patient has very few memories of this time, but claims to have been frequently ill. The kinesiologist finds an intolerance of sugar and wheat; all substances tested in the hand.
	AK Test Results: indicates generalized hypertonicity as a sign of maximum stress burdening. This can be balanced by vitamin B3, indicating a liver disorder.
	Wheat intolerance is revealed, also intolerance to all cow's milk products, rye, and carrots; however, this is only found when the foods are tested on the tongue. There is no reaction when the foods are tested by holding them in the hand.

but had no success!" This is not surprising. The application of every method, including that of kinesiology, requires correct indications and exact implementation to obtain meaningful results. For further information, please consult the International Medical Society for Applied Kinesiology (for address, see p. 139). All future references to muscle testing will imply the procedure utilised by AK in the medical field.

Kinesiology is not the same as AK! And not all kinesiologists know what they are talking about

AK Testing Application

AK testing is based on a change in muscle response. This means that we consciously expose the system—the "human being"—to stress and examine how the system responds. The response is visible and perceptible through the muscle test. These stresses can come from all fields of the "triad of health" and can be structural, mechanical, chemical, or emotional. The chemical side is of the greatest relevance with allergies.

Goodheart discovered that chemical substances such as medications, but also minerals, trace elements, and vitamins, can lead to temporary changes in the muscle test. The same also applies to foods, various allergens, and chemicals, so that their influence on the body becomes immediately visible and perceptible through the muscle test. Provocation and "trial treatment" with varying substances is referred to as challenge.

Whether a substance is classified as tolerated, therapeutically helpful, or not tolerated depends on the result of the muscle test. In accordance with the above classification—normotonic, weak, hypertonic—every measure that brings the muscle test to the biologically correct state of reaction can be considered therapeutically beneficial. On the other hand, everything that weakens the muscle or places it under stress (i. e., makes it hypertonic) is classified as not beneficial, burdening, or not tolerated. This means there is a fundamental difference between a change in the muscle reaction from normotonic to weak and a change in the opposite direction.

> Every measure that leads a muscle to a biologically correct response is therapeutically beneficial.

What Makes a Muscle Weak, What Makes it Strong?
When a previously strong muscle is weakened by a substance, it is to be assumed that this substance is not beneficial to the body. This could be a food, illness-causing agents in the environment, heavy metal, medication, or many other things. This test result is the fundamental principle in recognizing intolerances and allergies.

The second possibility, a weak muscle that becomes strong through the administration of various substances from all fields of medicine, is in keeping with the expected positive reaction to the right medication. This tells us whether the chosen homeopathic medications, vitamin, trace element, mineral, phyto-therapeutic substance, and of course allopathic medications, are beneficial within the investigation in question. Muscle testing does not replace the necessity of assessing prescribed medications, which clearly remains the responsibility of the investigating doctor.

When investigating allergies or intolerances, it is also important that the substances in question—allergens—are tested through contact with the mucous membrane or the skin. This means that foods, and also food supplements such as minerals, trace elements, and vitamins, are tested on the tongue. Creams and ointments are tested on the skin; volatile substances can be inhaled. Only in this way is the highest possible degree of accuracy of the test guaranteed. All other methods of kinesiological testing, for example, where the muscle test is applied with foods held in the hand, or indeed where the patient simply formulates or thinks about the food, are inadequate, open to wide margins of error, and do not comply with the high medical standards necessary to make a diagnosis.

Table 9 Muscles and Their Link to Organ Systems, Disorders and Nutrients

Muscle	Organ	Disorder	Nutrient
Front Thigh Muscle (quadriceps or rectus femoris)	Small Intestine	Dysbiosis, Allergy	Calcium, Vitamin C
Hip Abductor/ Flexor (tensor fasciae latae	Large Intestine	Anaemia	Iron, Vitamin B12, intestinal symbionts (probiotics)
Large pectoral muscle—breastbone (pectoralis sternalis)	Liver	Detoxification	Vitamin A, Bitter Substances, Foods
Large pectoral muscle—collar bone (pectoralis clavicularis)	Stomach	Acid–Base Balance	Zinc, Base Powder
Inner Thigh Muscle (sartorius)	Adrenal Glands	Hormone Balance	Vitamin C, Vitamin B6, Zinc
Rotatory Cuff (infraspinatus)	Thymus Gland	Immune System	Zinc, Copper, Vitamin A, Vitamin C

Experience has also shown that individual muscles have connections to organs and meridian systems of Chinese medicine. Thus conclusions can also be drawn about these organ systems by means of individual muscle responses.

The possibilities for applying AK in the medical field are very diverse. The following are important for our investigations:

- Recognizing response state
- Determining biochemical reaction of an allergy or intolerance
- Determining dysbiosis, parasitosis
- Testing of medications for level of tolerance
- Testing of orthomolecular substances
- Food testing
- Testing of material, e. g. for tooth replacement or dental work
- Testing of hormone balance
- Testing of chronic inflammation foci and focal disorders

Response State as a Stress Marker in AK Testing

We frequently encounter situations where patients have completely overloaded their regulatory system and display a generalized hypertonic state (= hypertonic muscle test response) affecting all muscles. We refer to this as "generalized hypertonicity." In terms of Selye's stress response, this corresponds to the phase of increased adaptation. Generalized hypertonicity is often a sign of regulatory rigidity in people suffering from allergies.

If a non-tolerated food triggers a temporary weakness in the AK muscle test, this is not just a transitory change, but provides important information about the body's regulatory capacity and the priority of the intolerance for the person being tested.

Allergy/Intolerance

At the start, a so-called "allergy screening" is carried out, in which various mediator substances, such as histamine or kinin, are tested for their effect. Should these lead to a change in the result of the muscle test, then an allergy or intolerance is to be assumed. This screening is then followed by testing of individual allergens.

Dysbiosis (Candida)/Parasite Infestations

We can now move on to dysbiosis (candidiasis) and/or parasite infestation of the digestive system and the body. AK is an outstanding supplement to the sensitive Mayr diagnostics. With Mayr diagnostics, we can recognize the effects of a food intolerance, allergy, or dysbiosis in the digestive system, and we can derive the exact cause by means of the muscle test. This enables quick identification of the appropriate medication.

Testing of Medications

Since there are always a number of problems and burdens, especially in the case of those suffering from allergies or chronic illnesses, administration of medication that tests well and is therefore individually well

---

Patient History

Patient G.D., female, age 58

Symptoms: for 32 years, following pregnancy, itching eczema on the legs, cracks in skin, chapped skin, weeping, partially bloody secretions, erysipeloid several times, various allergy tests were negative. Early retirement on account of incapacity to work.

Mayr Diagnostics: distended small and large intestines, liver congestion, chapped tongue, radix edema.
AK Test Results: generalized hypertonicity, yeast infestation.
Food Test Results: intolerance to several cereal grains as well as cow's milk products and yeast. Positive reaction to base powder, calcium, vitamin C, and copper.

Mayr Therapy: After a 4-week out-patient Mayr therapy, applying the candida diet, pronounced improvement, eczema diminishing, clear improvement regarding the allergy. After 3 months continuation of Mayr therapy and further avoidance of the nontolerated foods, signs of the intolerance are diminishing, pronounced improvement of the skin. Only wheat, yeast, and cow's milk products are still not tolerated. After 5 months: only wheat and cow's milk products are not tolerated. General well-being, legs completely healed, skin symptom free.

---

tolerated takes on particular importance. Muscle testing can quickly demonstrate that many of the common (allopathic) medications, although they contain relevant active substances, actually lead to a weakening in the muscle test, due to many fillers and binders that are not declared on the label. Consequently, these cannot be prescribed. Determining which medications either cause allergies or intensify already existing allergies is therefore quickly and easily possible with AK l.

Due to the fact that the substances being tested are always brought into contact with the mucous membrane of a patient during testing, this method is considerably more sensitive than most common procedures. However, neglecting this necessity opens the door to errors and incorrect test results. Substances that are only tested in the hand or in the package will not necessarily produce a correct test result.

Orthomolecular Substances
In the field of orthomolecular medications, the body's own substances are used both as prevention and therapy. The minerals, trace elements, enzymes, proteins, vitamins, or amino acids used, high doses of which are sometimes administered, should be given as pure substances whenever possible because of the considerations previously mentioned.

The advantage offered by AK is the immediate response of the patient to the orthomolecular substance to be therapeutically administered. The question of antagonism—for example in mineral balance (zinc–copper, iron–copper, calcium–magnesium)—can also be quickly included in therapeutic considerations and therapy can be adapted quickly and effectively to changing requirements.

Orthomolecular substances selection will be discussed later (see pp. 112).

Food Testing
This is an essential part of AK testing. If an allergy, intolerance, or dysbiosis has been discovered, a food test is always carried out. Important and frequently poorly tolerated foods are cow's milk products, wheat,

and yeast. These, at least, should be tested. For Mayr therapy, all foods to be consumed during therapy must be tested (see p. 103).

Testing of Materials

Tolerance of tooth-replacement material is a frequently raised question. Investigating this remains the domain of the dentist, as only a dentist can correctly assess the situation. However, dental material producing poor AK test results is frequently found in cases of chronic burdening such as dysbiosis and allergies. In these cases, an acceptable solution must be found in cooperation with the dentist.

Hormone Balance

Diagnosing and treating hormone imbalance requires knowledge of biochemical and molecular-biological connections. Here, too, AK offers a quick overview of the functional connections of hormonal balancing. An allergy that has existed for a considerable length of time practically always leads to hormonal exhaustion. Here we think again of Selye, the father of stress research, and list once again his three organ systems that are always affected in cases of stress:

- Stomach – acid-base balance
- Thymus Gland – immune system
- Adrenal glands – hormone system

AK can provide ideal reinforcement for hormone balancing. In people with long-standing allergies, the adrenal glands in particular are likely to be exhausted. Appropriately tested substances to stimulate the adrenal glands often produce a breakthrough in therapy.

Focal Disorders

In medicine, the significance of focal disorders is now widely accepted. A focal disorder is an area of tissue that does not participate in the normal regulation of the body. However, it cannot always be clearly determined whether or not a suspicious region (scar, tooth) acts as an irritant. AK, with therapy localisation, lets us quickly determine whether or not the suspicious region needs to be treated. In addition, we can investigate which therapeutic measures are effective and also how long the success of the therapy lasts, by retesting at (ir)regular intervals an area of irritation that has been found.

Supplementary Testing

Clearly, AK is not a replacement for necessary laboratory testing, but is a valuable supplement to it. AK is also a useful tool in deciding which laboratory tests are most relevant.

Supplementary to the previous examinations, individual parameters in the laboratory can indicate an allergy or intolerance. Among these are the levels of enzymes, such as diamine oxidase

> AK is the quickest method for a doctor to determine the most effective therapy and to test its results.

(measurement for the breakdown of histamine). Of particular importance is the determination of vitamins, minerals, and trace elements in whole blood. The reason for this is that important minerals occur in higher levels inside the cell than outside it. Zinc is particularly relevant here, but also copper, vitamin B6, and vitamin C are parameters in histamine intolerance.

Burdening with heavy metals such as mercury or lead can also be proven by mobilization and elimination via the urine. This is to be recommended, particularly in cases of chronic disorders, because heavy metals can block detoxification of the lymph and enzyme systems.

However, all laboratory examinations are only supplementary diagnostic measures and are recommended and carried out by the doctor in charge of treatment in each individual case.

Often, a patient is surprised by the muscle test response and asks, "What has just happened?" Indeed, how much higher is the motivation of patients to take the appropriate medications or to carry out the recommended procedure, when they have has experienced the result of the test? This is one of the enormous advantages of AK. Through muscle testing, patients notice very quickly how they react to various influences. A patient can feel the weakness of a muscle, triggered by the allergen, and also the strengthening, pain-relieving effects of different medications. This is also important for the doctor treating the patient, because this means that a large proportion of the motivation to carry out the necessary therapy results from the method itself.

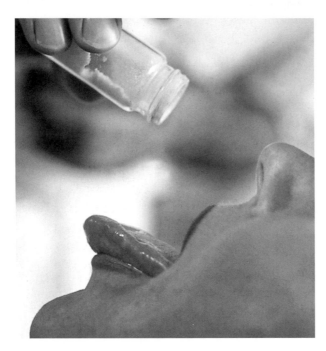

Fig. 14 Allergies can also be determined by medication testing, referred to as "oral" challenge.

Allergy Therapy Opportunities

The goal of allergy therapy is to achieve appropriate immune system response. When we consider the wide variety of possible influences, then various starting points are both possible and necessary in therapy. What is important here is to both know and identify the triggering factors as accurately as possible, in order to subsequently avoid them by temporarily refraining from contact with them.

Individual therapeutic measures are both necessary and important; however, effective therapy combines the widest range of possibilities in a complementary way that is tailored to the individual patient.

Therapy, of course, depends on the intensity and current state of symptoms. It is not our intent to create the impression that every acute allergic reaction is to be treated solely by Mayr therapy and the administration of minerals. Cases of acute or even life-threatening conditions require intensive medical intervention. This is not the objective of this discussion.

In the following, we are more interested in chronic symptoms for which a cause has not been clearly established. Symptoms that do not primarily suggest an allergy, such as joint disorders, are also included in the therapeutic considerations. Let us first take a look at the four columns of promising allergy therapy (see Fig. 15).

Prevention is Better than Cure
Part of the therapy lies in the avoidance of the triggering allergens. This is generally appreciated, but unfortunately is frequently the only preventive measure. As was shown in diagnostics, foods are more frequently involved in allergies than is generally assumed.

But avoiding misdigestion must also be mentioned as part of allergy prevention. Preventing an allergy-triggering situation involves a change in nutritional habits and way of life. This often includes "individual stress management," both of a physical and a spiritual—emotional—mental kind.

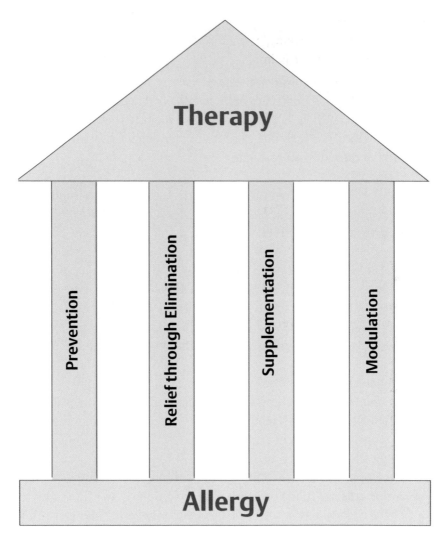

Fig. 15 The Four Columns of Allergy Therapy

Relieving the Immune System through Elimination of Disruptive Factors
This requires cleansing, detoxification, and elimination of everything disruptive. Only in this way can the immune system be restored to a state of normal response. As long as the body is full of toxic substances, this objective can only be partially achieved, with a subsequent return to the old pattern, often repeatedly.

Supplementation

of everything that is lacking, to enable the immune system to function biologically correctly. It is important to recognize that the absence of individual components endangers the optimal functioning of the entire immune system. We should mention, above all, minerals, trace elements, and vitamins that were needed in other places and are now no longer available in adequate amounts for the immune system.

Modulation

is the fine adjustment of the immune system on all levels of possible regulation. And it is individuality more than anything else that plays the decisive role. No two immune systems react in exactly the same way. Each is integrated within the individuality of the person.

For this reason, comprehensive allergy therapy must be individually designed and carried out as holistically as possible. Mayr therapy is meaningful in the long term in order to restore the body's regulatory capacity and to actively improve the state of health.

Basic Principles of Modern Mayr Medicine

Modern F.X. Mayr medicine is a holistic method. Based on Mayr diagnostics, it applies the therapy principles of rest and simplification, cleansing, training and supplementation in an individually designed therapy program. Mayr therapy improves all organ functions and increases quality of life.

It is important that the therapy addresses the causes of allergies or intolerances. There are many direct links between digestive health and allergies, which underscores the need to make essential changes in nutritional habits. Mayr therapy is the first step toward this goal.

Key Concepts of F.X. Mayr Therapy™

Mayr therapy takes time. As a natural therapy, it does not live up to the "turbo charged" expectations of our fast-moving age. Mayr therapy means replacing current habits with new ones, as well as relearning and maintaining healthy eating habits. It means taking the time to reprogram our autonomic (vegetative) nervous system. Achieving lasting improvements requires more than carrying out a one-time Mayr therapy; it requires recognizing basic principles and acting accordingly. A meaningful Mayr therapy lasts 3 to 4 weeks. Shorter therapies are possible and can be important measures; however, they do not constitute comprehensive regeneration. We will come back to this point in the section on therapy strategies.

Mayr therapy is also the observation of rhythms, both small and large. Everything in life is movement and therefore rhythmic. Regeneration and recuperation need these rhythms: day–night rhythm, organ clock, weekly rhythm, and annual rhythm. These rhythms keep this miracle called "human being" going. Activity alternates with relaxation. Both exist alongside each other. If we overtax ourselves occasionally, we can draw on compensatory mechanisms to balance it out. But not indefinitely. Overtaxing our rhythms always reduces minerals, trace elements, and vitamins. This points to the importance of regular phases of regeneration in accordance with Mayr principles.

Mayr therapy is not only physical cleansing, but also a mental and emotional/spiritual process. During Mayr therapy, participants abstain voluntarily and consciously reduce the quantity and type of foods they take in. Voluntary participation is key for therapy to be successful; without it, therapy will fail. As Mayr doctors, we will inform, guide, and motivate our patients, but we will not "persuade" them and never force them.

For example, we have recognized with fructose intolerance that its biochemical background effects emotions. This applies indirectly to many situations of intestinal autointoxification. People who are prepared to conduct emotional and mental cleansing will discover ways and possibilities they have never before considered. Along the way, there are many obstacles to be overcome in the form of emotional crises, but then the head becomes clearer, we can think freely, creativity returns, mood stabilizes, and rediscovering our inner strength becomes easier.

> Unless Mayr therapy is carried out willingly, the patient will not become healthier, but increasingly ill.

Allergies have to do with boundaries and how these are dealt with. Whether it is the intestines acting as the boundary between the inside and outside world, or the lungs or skin; allergies always impact our personal boundaries. Rudolf Steiner once explained it thus: "A person suffering from an allergy melts into his/her environment." Addressing this issue can sometimes lead to decisive improvements in symptoms.

Mayr Therapy is Accomplished by the Patient!

No doctor can meet the expectation of a patient who says "I am ill, make me healthy!" without the patient's active participation and patience. To begin with, this is not how "healing" works. Mayr doctors view themselves more as a companion, a mountain guide—as Mayr called it—for climbing the mountain of health. And if health really is an independent strength, as mentioned at the beginning, then we, as Mayr doctors, will promote, uncover, and utilize this strength in our patients in every possible way. This means treating our patient as partners who will take responsibility for their own health. Our patients must assume responsibility for their   physical as well as for their mental and emotional/spiritual recovery.

Patient History	**Patient G.G., female, age 21**
	Symptoms: recurring bladder inflammation, frequent antibiotic therapy, depression for 3 months, known allergies to household dust, cats, birch, and ash trees.
	Mayr Diagnostics: inflamed small intestine, slight liver congestion, radix edema.
	AK Test Results: generalized hypertonicity, histamine intolerance, parasite infestation.
	In the food test, intolerance to cow's milk products.
	Mayr Therapy: After a 4-week out-patient Mayr therapy, there is clear improvement; mood is very good, no bladder disorder whatsoever. No parasite infestation, continued intolerance to cow's milk products. Continued avoidance of certain foods.
	Check-up after 3 months, continued freedom from symptoms, no inflammation whatsoever, depression disappeared. Of cow's milk products, butter is now tolerated, indicating onset of improvement.

Understanding this fundamental consideration is key. The practical implementation methods described in the following are to be viewed as more than the mechanics of therapy: they must be understood as the beginning of individualized and personal reorientation of nutritional habits and way of life.

Therapeutic Principles of Mayr Therapy: Rest and Simplification, Cleansing, Training, Substitution

Mayr therapy is a form of treatment that appropriately applies the therapeutic principles of rest and simplification, cleansing, training, and supplementation. These principles must, of course, be individually structured and applied concurrently and over an adequate period. Parameters determined during the initial examination using Mayr diagnostics serve as the foundation for this therapy.

Rest and Simplification

Rest and simplification in this context means focusing on the essentials. It is one of the oldest healing principles of nature and medicine. A sick animal will temporarily reduce or cease its food supply and withdraw. Bed rest is recommended for feverish illness. Injuries often require resting or immobilizing, and in the case of a broken leg, the leg is placed in splints or a cast to enable healing in peace. The digestive system cannot be placed in splints or in a cast. Rest for the digestive system is achieved by reducing and simplifying food supply and by practising healthy eating habits.

Rest and simplification can take place at different levels of intensity, depending on the individual's diagnostic criteria. The degree to which a patient willingly cooperates is, of course, also of significance.

Individual Possibilities for Rest and Simplification:
- Tea/water fasting
- Milk diet
- Extended milk diet
- Mild Clearing Diet
- Special forms

In recent years, the significance of mild forms of therapy has increased. Our restorative capacity is impaired due to many factors. Our lifestyle and nutritional situation, but also the enormous increase in stress reduce our ability to compensate and react appropriately to further challenges. It is therefore frequently more beneficial to choose a form of therapy that is somewhat milder, but that can be carried out over a longer period.

Resting through Continual Repetition

Resting necessitates a certain degree of simplification and monotony. This simplification is a fundamentally important healing factor. In the most intensive form of fasting, tea or water fasting, simplification is provided for by only consuming liquids. Later, simplification is achieved by always consuming the same foods during therapy. For example, one milk product is chosen and consumed throughout the entire therapy. It is not recommended to alternate between milk, yogurt, sour milk, or other products, or to eat milk in the morning and yogurt for lunch. The same applies to the bread roll. The Mild Clearing Diet also constitutes a degree of simplification, if we compare its choice and preparation of foods with the mixture of ingredients in our everyday meals. Rest and simplification

---

Patient History	**Patient A.B., female, age 31**

Symptoms: significantly overweight, 85 kg at a height of 175 cm. Really wants to lose weight, eats little, exercises and sweats well when doing so, drinks plenty; her weight nevertheless increases. Laboratory tests, including hormone level, reveal nothing really noticeable. Patient insists on strict fasting to lose weight.

Mayr Diagnostics: clear signs of exhaustion despite overweight, small and large intestine sluggish and congested, diminishment vitality, sensitive kidney reflex zones.

Mayr Therapy: Recommendation to start with Mild Clearing Diet and to observe many periods of rest. Despite this advice, patient begins with strict fasting for 1 week, resulting in a mere 1 kg weight loss (patient frustrated). Abdominal results are worsening, the patient is retaining water, short-term increase in weight. The situation is subsequently explained to the patient in detail once more. Treatment is now continued with the Mild Clearing Diet. This results in immediate improvement. Sense of well-being increases, satisfactory elimination; after 6 weeks, patient feels completely well, her weight is 70 kg.

also occurs through the selection and preparation of foods during Mayr therapy. (Contact the Golf Hotel Health Center at the address at the end of the book for more information about the Mild Clearing Diet).

A Stale White Bread Roll as Therapeutic Measure

We want to offer rest and simplification to the digestive system as the uppermost and most important principle of therapy. This means that, for a certain period, we will only provide it with foods that demand a minimum of digestive performance. Among these are all-purpose flour or white flour.

We would like to emphasize that the value of a white bread roll during Mayr therapy is not in providing vital substances, but as a "chewing trainer." It would be completely wrong and against the healing principles of Mayr therapy if a whole-grain (whole meal) roll were used for therapy. This puts too great a strain on the digestive system and is inappropriate for Mayr therapy. The ideal during therapy is an approximately 2 or 3-day-old bread roll made from super-finely ground white flour (e.g. all-purpose, cake, or pastry flour).

The Mild Clearing Diet focuses on easy digestibility in the choice and preparation of food. The rest and simplification factor is, of course, not as intensive here, but considering everyday life and the necessity of a mild form of therapy, it is exactly the right therapy for many patients.

Cultivating healthy eating habits is, of course, not only good training for everyday life, but ensures optimal digestion. Observing a daily rhythm, where the evening meal should be the smallest and most easily digestible, is also important in this context.

The Principle of Rest and Simplification

We must view rest and simplification in a comprehensive sense and not only in relation to the digestive system. If we assume that many people have to cope with enormous stress, then everything should be done to combat this stress.

Selye refers to rest, recuperation, and relaxation as the most important measures against stress. The sources of stress are irrelevant— be they emotional problems, work-related problems, or personal problems, chemical stresses through allergies or mineral deficiencies, or structural stresses (e. g., because of a misaligned jawbone or faulty bite). Anything that reduces digestive performance must be avoided while eating—reading the newspaper, listening to the radio, watching TV, talking on the telephone, working at the computer, eating at work or eating "on the run." All of these activities influence digestive performance.

> When we eat while physically, mentally, or emotionally overtired, we will not be able to convert even the best foods properly.

Rest and simplification also means consciously switching off and distancing ourselves from "bad news" broadcast by the many channels of modern news communication. Leaving the television set and the radio switched off, working less, taking more breaks to rest, consciously switching off, and inner reflection are all of enormous help in this respect.

Rest and Exercise
Rest and simplification also includes reducing physical activity. Today many people are seized by running, cycling, tennis, golf, or fitness "fever." Sensibly conducted, exercise reinforces the regeneration process, but only if it observes the principle of rest and simplification. Recommended are types of exercise that serve the gradual combustion of fat such as gentle forms of stretching, isometrics, yoga, walking, hiking, cycling, and golf.

A simple test of the individual's lactate threshold can provide good information to determine the appropriate level of exercise for each individual. The results of this test are useful in preventing overtaxation during exercise, which creates an acid metabolic process. On the other hand, strict physical rest will be necessary from time to time, to enable comprehensive regeneration.

The manner and intensity of rest and simplification depends on the therapeutic environment. There is a difference between carrying out a Mayr therapy on an in-patient or an out-patient basis. What is important is that all the individual measures together do not result in overtaxing.

This applies both during Mayr therapy and in everyday life. During Mayr therapy, overtaxing leads to unpleasant reactions; in everyday life, it constitutes the beginning of intestinal autointoxification.

Cleansing

Cleansing means cleaning the body. For this we use the intestines as well as all other possibilities of excreting toxins, for example the kidneys, skin, lungs, or the so-called "emergency valves."

As was shown earlier in this book, misdigestion produces a series of toxic substances and waste products in the intestines. Since these impair normal functioning of the intestines, elimination of toxins and waste products is also impaired. Instead, toxins are stored, first in the intestines and later also in connective tissue, a process referred to as tissue clogging. As a result, physiological self-cleansing of the digestive system, and subsequently of the entire body, is disrupted.

F.X. Mayr worked for a long time in Carlsbad, a healing resort in today's Czech Republic, which has been known for its healing hot springs and sulphuric mud for more than 500 years. There, he recognized the cleansing effect of the Carlsbad water. It is a mixture of Glauber's salt, Epsom (bitter) salts, and sodium bicarbonate. Today, we mostly use Epsom salts or Glauber's salt, since Carlsbad water is not obtainable. One level teaspoon of the salt is dissolved in a quarter of a liter (4 cups) of warm water and is drunk in the morning on an empty stomach. This loosens the contents of the intestines slowly from the top to the bottom and enables their elimination. One of the most important effects of Epsom salts in this context is the retention of water in the intestines. This is essential for successfully cleansing them. It does not make sense to increase the amount of Epsom salts following the motto "more is better." This can lead to unpleasant reactions and is not helpful. Epsom salts or Glauber's salt often produce intensive emptying of the bowels. To avoid overtaxing here also, the F.X. passage effervescent salts—which have a gentler effect—can be taken instead.

A further effect of Epsom salts is its stimulation of the liver–gall bladder activity. This indirectly stimulates intestinal peristalsis, which is important for elimination.

Elimination of Toxins

Intestinal cleansing is an important step in our "cleansing" strategy. The inner surface of our intestines is the size of a football field, and an area of this size cannot be cleansed taking Epsom salts only once or twice. Continual cleansing is therefore necessary, above all the elimination of mobilized toxins. If these toxins are not eliminated in the proper period of time, the body will attempt to reabsorb them, which can produce unpleasant symptoms of reintoxification. This easily occurs at the beginning of therapy, because the body first has to relearn how to eliminate concentrated toxins. Appropriate supportive measures are frequently necessary (see p. 86). However, once cleansing of the intestines is in full swing, the intestines themselves can again function as an organ of elimination.

The second step is cleansing of the lymph fluids and the blood with subsequent cleansing of the tissue. This phase is important for the long-term effect of Mayr therapy, because it removes metabolic toxins from the tissue they have been stored in. This process obviously takes more time and that is why Mayr therapy lasts 3 to 4 weeks.

Avoiding Reintoxification

We can trust that elimination of stored toxins follows a well thought-out hierarchy. The body differentiates between healthy and sick, between what is useful and what has been stored. An act of cleansing is triggered, unnecessary waste products are broken down; however, essential tissue is not destroyed. The intestines, increasingly cleansed, function increasingly better as therapy progresses and produce a suction effect for waste products, which mobilizes and eliminates them. However, in all phases of cleansing, overtaxing of the elimination system can occur. This creates a backlog of toxins and reabsorption. The resulting reintoxification can cause severe reactions from time to time. These are unpleasant but mostly completely harmless. With appropriate rein- forcement of elimination, they abate very quickly (see pp. 102).

With allergies, many of the toxins that are temporarily deposited in the tissue and then mobilized are acid and protein components. These can- not simply be eliminated from the body. Acids first have to be neutral- ized by means of bases, and protein must also be appropriately metab- olized. The liver is responsible for all these tasks. It is our "main metabolic organ" for detoxification. Supporting the liver will therefore be an important part of Mayr therapy.

No Detoxification without Water

Water constitutes 60 to 70% of our body. Water is absolutely *the* me- dium of metabolism. Many metabolic processes take place in a watery environment, above all the transport of toxins. Anything transported via the lymph or the blood must first be made "water soluble." Even fat, which normally cannot be dissolved in water, is transported in bod- ily fluids by being bound to various substances. Absorbing water is the task of the intestines; filtering the blood and producing urine as an elimination product is the task of the kidneys. Many unusable sub- stances, but also the metabolic toxins, are emitted with the urine. The kidneys are so well supplied with blood that their daily filter capacity would fill a bath-tub. It is therefore important to drink sufficient quan- tities of clear liquids in everyday life, but particularly important during Mayr therapy.

Our metabolism cannot produce the performance demanded of it with- out the necessary quantities of liquid. It is recommended that a person with a body weight of approximately 70 kg drink 3 l per day, 4 l, and more if the weight is higher (4 cups of water for every 50 lbs. of body weight; for example, a person weighing 175 lbs. should drink 14 or more cups of water daily).

> Every Mayr therapy is also a drinking cure.

Some people are initially amazed by these quantities, particularly as very little is drunk in normal everyday life, and even more so when only the following are considered as liquids:

- good spring water
- noncarbonated mineral water
- briefly brewed, mild herbal teas
- clear vegetable broths

Most importantly, all varieties of fruit juices, soft drinks, carbonated beverages, energy drinks, as well as alcohol and coffee are not classified as appropriate liquids in this context. It is also important that liquids are consumed continually throughout the day, above all between meals.

Before and after meals, a one hour break should be observed for drinking, because during meals, we need concentrated, efficient digestive juices, both during the Mayr therapy and in our everyday lives. Drinking during meals, or shortly before or after meals, dilutes these digestive juices and thus reduces digestive efficiency, which is so important at this time.

Preparation of Tea

Nearly all herbal teas that reinforce metabolic processes, detoxification and cleansing of the blood, bodily fluids and the liver are suitable. Since herbal teas are primarily used as a way of supplying the body with liquid, they are prepared in a somewhat modified way.

> Briefly steep teas (30-60 sec) to let the water takes on the aroma, but not any undesired active herb substances.

Pour hot water over a small amount of the tea (about as much 3 fingers can hold for 1 liter/quart of water). Let it steep for 30-60 seconds and strain. The tea is now ready for drinking (hot or cooled down). Such brief brewing allows the aromatic herb substances to go into the tea, but is not enough time for the herbs' pharmacological effects to become too intensive. Of course, some of the effect of the herb is always present, if large quantities of tea are drunk.

The Following Teas Are Very Suitable during Mayr Therapy:
- St. John's Wort (Rose of Sharon)
- Horsetail
- Sage
- Rosemary
- Lemon Balm
- Melilot (Sweet Clover)
- Thyme
- Yarrow
- Anserine (Wormseed)
- Fennel

Of course, tea mixtures can also be prepared. It is always advisable to alternate the teas used. Green tea is also acceptable. Black tea should be drunk in only modest quantities, if at all, because it has been fermented.

The Following Teas Are Not Beneficial:
- Chamomile: reduces the activity of the intestines and should be drunk only in case of acute gastro-intestinal disorders.
- Peppermint: is much too pungent and intensive during the Mayr therapy.
- Red fruit and blossom teas (e. g. hibiscus, rose hip): are too acidic. The more basic herbal teas are given preference during Mayr therapy.

Unfortunately, it is mostly the non-beneficial teas that are offered in restaurants. It is better to avoid these teas and drink only water. Should there be no other possibility of obtaining tea, consumption of the above teas will not put therapy success at risk, as long as they are brewed for only a short time and drunk in very small quantities.

Clear vegetable broth is also an ideal drink as it contains many valuable mineral substances from the vegetables.

Recipe for Clear Vegetable Broth/Base Broth
Use organically grown or unsprayed vegetables wherever possible. Root vegetables give a stronger taste so that it is preferable to use carrots, turnips, root celery, stick celery, fennel, parsnip, and potatoes. Quality and combination determine the taste.

It is not necessary to salt this broth since many root vegetables have a slightly salty taste. The vegetables remaining after the broth has been

Recipe	Use one-third vegetables to two-thirds water. Cut vegetables into small pieces (a food processor can speed up this step) and place into cold water. Add fresh herbs, a bay leaf, pepper corns (optional), a few juniper berries, and a pinch of nutmeg. Simmer, rather than boil, for approximately 30 to 40 minutes. Strain through a fine sieve, cool to a comfortable temperature, and drink in sips.

strained can be placed in cold water and used again. This second, or even third, brew is used in the preparation of base soups and sauces.

The addition of vegetable soup seasoning is possible and it intensifies the taste; however, in the case of an allergy or intolerance, this ready-made product as well as all soup ingredients must be tested for tolerance. If tolerated, instant clear vegetable broth is an alternative for people who work or when underway.

The Lungs as Organs of Elimination

The lungs are responsible for the exchange of gaseous substances. Whereas the surface area of the digestive system corresponds approximately to that of a football field, the surface area of the lungs amounts to approximately 80 m^2 (about 800sq ft). In our lungs, oxygen is taken in via inhaled air and carbon dioxide is emitted through exhalation. Carbon dioxide is an end product of the body's metabolic processes. It is transported to the lungs via the blood and then exhaled.

We can expand on the function of the lungs to the extent that all gaseous substances can be eliminated via the lungs. We have already met hydrogen as a fermentation product with fructose intolerance. In addition, there is a whole range of other fermentation and putrefaction products that likewise have to be eliminated via the lungs. Increased excretion via the lungs often becomes noticeable as "bad breath," which is mostly noticed by other people and not by the person involved.

Increased but not over-exaggerated breathing promotes elimination of these gaseous substances. In addition, exhalation of carbon dioxide is the fastest regulatory process for acid–base balance. Exercise promotes breathing activity and therefore detoxification. Exercise is therefore important during Mayr therapy. However, particularly in the case of allergies involving the lungs, attention must be paid to avoiding overexertion.

Bad breath during Mayr therapy is a clear indication of ongoing detoxification.

The Skin

The skin with all its glands is also an important organ of elimination. Liquid is regularly evaporated via the skin, thus providing an opportunity for emitting toxins. Of course, perspiration—whether provoked actively through exercise or passively, e.g. in a sauna, steam bath, or any other way—is also a valve for the emission of toxins. In addition, the skin is a reflex organ, meaning that internal organs are represented on the skin surface. These many different kinds of reflex zones provide us with diagnostic indications of disorders of the internal organs. At the same time, we can influence internal organs and their function by treating these reflex zones.

Supportive Measures for Cleansing

It is important for Mayr therapy to utilize all possibilities of elimination. Even more importantly, the goal is to support some systems in order to relieve others. This can employ the following measures:

- Manual abdominal treatment by a Mayr doctor
- Enema
- Colon hydrotherapy
- Baths
- Kneipp applications
- Massages
- Inhalations

Manual Abdominal Treatment by a Mayr Doctor

The manual abdominal treatment is carried out by specially trained Mayr doctors. It is an essential, indispensable part of every Mayr therapy. (Implementation and effect of this important component of Mayr therapy are described in more detail on p. 97.) Here, only the areas of detoxification and cleansing are mentioned. Manual abdominal treatment mobilizes the contents of the intestines, which can then be eliminated more easily, or in some cases can only then be eliminated. It therefore directly supports intestinal cleansing. Manual abdominal treatment also promotes transport of congested lymph from the region of the intestines (decongesting the radix edema) and of venous blood from the abdomen.

Enema

In case of difficulties with elimination, the use of an enema is always worthwhile. The objective is to loosen the contents of the large intestine with warm water so that it can be excreted. The water that has been inserted into the large intestine, should not be retained, but should immediately leave the intestines again. This loosens stored, impacted fecal matter, dilutes toxins, and cleanses the large intestines. Enemas have proven particularly useful in cases of headaches, migraine, insufficient elimination via the intestines, and both initial and late reactions during Mayr therapy.

Colon Hydrotherapy

Colon hydrotherapy is an intensification of the enema. While enemas can cleans the last third of the large intestine, colon-hydrotherapy can rinse the entire large intestine. What is important here is that a trained person treats the abdomen simultaneously or, even better, that a manual abdominal treatment is carried out by a Mayr doctor during colon hydrotherapy.

Colon-Hydrotherapy is not always appropriate. In cases of allergy, It can even cause a worsening of symptoms.

With colon hydrotherapy, it is critical to avoid an "open ICV" arising. What does this mean? At the point where the small and large intestines join, there is a functional valve, the Bauhin valve or ICV (ileocecal valve).

This opens to allow the contents of the intestines to flow from the small intestine into the large intestine. When closed, it prevents the contents of the large intestine from flowing back into the small intestine. If this region becomes chronically irritated, which frequently occurs with allergy symptoms, it remains functionally open. If colon hydrotherapy is carried out in such cases, the contents of the large intestine are rinsed back into the small intestine. The result is that the patient is in a worse condition after colon hydrotherapy than before. This demonstrates that it makes very little sense to apply even something that is helpful without due consideration. Colon hydrotherapy is not a fixed component of Mayr therapy. It is carried out in individual cases in accordance with certain indications, where it can be exceptionally helpful and result in the rapid diminishing of reintoxification reactions. There is also very little point in carrying out colon hydrotherapy in "blocks of ten."

Baths—Kneipp Applications

Particular attention must be paid to the interplay between the lungs and the skin, especially in the case of allergy symptoms (see p. 90). There are many ways of improving the skin's metabolism, including baths, Kneipp applications, and massages. A great many acids are also eliminated via the skin. The question arises as to whether the "acid mantle" of the skin really is a protection or whether it indicates the necessity and the possibility of eliminating acids via the skin. Whatever the case, acids irritate the skin.

Toxins can escape via the skin by means of appropriate baths. Bases or herbal essences should be added to the bath water, the temperature of which can be gradually increased. The simplest additions are natural soaps (e. g., Marseille soap, olive oil soap), baking soda, base powder, or ready-made base bath-mixtures.

Kneipp alternating hot-cold rinses and baths also stimulate detoxification, not only via the skin. They are simple measures that can produces enormous increases in well-being.

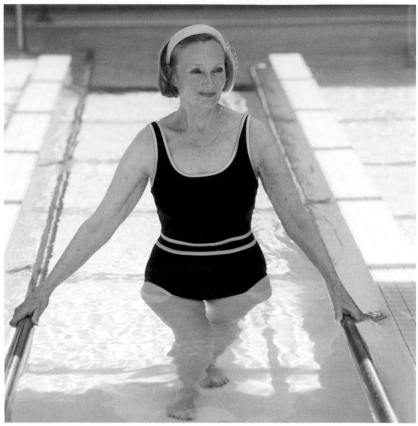

Fig. 16 "Kneipping" simply does you good.

Massages

Massages are effective primarily because they increase blood circulation and stimulate lymph drainage, as long as they are not carried out for the muscle–tendon area. For example, manual lymph drainage gently, but effectively stimulates lymph circulation. Since we know that the lymph performs immune functions, massages are considered important measures, and not only for allergies. Elimination can also be stimulated with reflex-zone massages, for example, for the foot reflex zones.

Inhalations

Inhalations using sea water or salt water can be useful for improving lung function. Various medicinal substances can be added such as essential oils, homoeopathic medications, or expectorant substances. Testing of these substances to make sure they are tolerated is important.

Training

The objective of training is to relearn healthy eating habits. This is the key ingredient for long-term success of any Mayr therapy.

We described at the beginning of this book how not paying attention to healthy eating habits leads to misdigestion, intestinal autointoxification, and allergies. The objective of training is to enable lasting changes in this area. Changing eating habits is frequently the most difficult and the most prolonged, because it calls into question 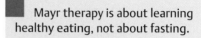 Mayr therapy is about learning healthy eating, not about fasting. many habits we have grown fond of. Nevertheless, or perhaps exactly for this reason, we need to assure that training is consistently practised during Mayr therapy.

Training involves:
- Eating slowly.
- Chewing and insalivating well at every meal. (Mayr himself described this as "souping." Food is chewed until it becomes a liquid mush of saliva and food.)
- Taking time to eat.
- During meals, avoiding everything that can reduce the production of saliva. This includes not drinking during meals, not letting yourself be distracted, for example by reading the newspaper, watching TV, listening to the radio, or stressful conversations.
- Stopping eating when the food tastes best; this means when a gentle, pleasant feeling of satiation occurs.
  Giving the digestive system time to digest. This means no snacks between meals; intervals between meals should be about 4 to 5 hours.

- Making the evening meal the smallest, the foods chosen for it the most easily digestible, and eating as early as possible. (Here, too, attention must be paid to good chewing and insalivating.)
- Paying attention to tolerance and easy digestibility in choice and preparation of food.
- Drinking sufficient quantities of clear liquid between meals (spring water, noncarbonated mineral water, herbal tea, clear vegetable broth,). No drinking during meals and 45 minutes before or after meals to avoid dilution of digestive juices
- Letting nothing and nobody detract you from practicing these measures.

These measures represent a profound change for most people and demand a certain amount of adjustment. Carrying them out in the desired intensity will only be possible during Mayr therapy, but we all need to implement this training repeatedly in order to integrate at least some of the above habits into our daily lives. We can only consciously influence our digestion as long as the food is still in our mouth. We can deliberately eat slowly and chew well.

Learning new chewing and digestive habits is an essential component of Mayr therapy.

Once the food we eat has left our mouth, digestion proceeds unconsciously, autonomously. There is no way to say to the stomach, "digest better" or to tell the small intestine to move more.

Our eating habits were acquired in earliest childhood. Changing them later in life requires conscious effort. We need to replace old habits with new ones, and then continually train and repeat these new habits until they are fully established. This change has to be accomplished by everyone who undergoes Mayr therapy and it is crucial. It also distinguishes Mayr therapy from other diets and fasting constraints.

Relearning healthy eating habits is our own responsibility. Whether we eat quickly without adequate chewing, gulping down food, or whether we quietly chew with relish, enjoying the food to the fullest, is solely our decision. It is not the doctor who "makes" the patient healthy again;

each individual endeavours to become healthier by changing their behaviour. Thus each individual can be justifiably proud of their achievement and of having made an active effort to recuperate.

Manual Abdominal Treatment by a Mayr Doctor

Doctors can support a patient's endeavours to recuperate by carrying out the manual abdominal treatment. This treatment was developed by F.X. Mayr and is an indispensable part of every Mayr therapy. It is a soft, gentle, partially rhythmic and breathing-synchronous treatment of the abdominal region. The treatment is an ideal complement to and supports cleansing and training.

The manual abdominal treatment stimulates intestinal activity. Its gentle changes in pressure move the contents of the intestines along. It produces more effective absorption of intestinal contents and elimination of waste. The manual abdominal treatment improves blood circulation in the abdominal region. This enables blood and lymph fluid to be transported better and more quickly from congested and/or inflamed sections of the intestines and be replaced by fresh, oxygenated blood and "clean" lymph fluid. As congestion and inflammation recedes, any pain in this area also diminishes. The manual abdominal treatment also improves tonus, shape, and position of the organs of the digestive system.

Improved activity of the intestines faster transport, increased blood circulation, and reduction of polluted lymph causes the individual digestive organs to regain improved tonus and return to

> The manual abdominal treatment cleanses intestines, blood, and fluids.

occupying the places designated for them. They become more supple and can be shifted more easily. The condition of the entire abdomen approaches the characteristics of ideal health. In most cases it becomes smaller, more free of pain, and easily palpable. This positively impacts all body cells. Their tonus and therefore their function also improve.

The improved relationships in the abdominal region result in the toxins being passed on intensively to the intestines via the lymph and blood.

Patient History	**Patient R.K., female, age 51**
	Symptoms: patient comes to Mayr therapy following acute intestinal inflammation and antibiotic therapy, with yeast infection and proof of candidiasis in the intestines. She is afraid of strict fasting and further weight loss.
	Mayr Diagnostics: distended, extremely sluggish, tired intestines, liver congested, enlarged, signs of exhaustion. *AK Test Results*: candidiasis is confirmed, additional stress response to conventional anti-fungal medication. Biological preparations indicate good effectiveness. Pronounced exhaustion of hormone system.
	Mayr Therapy: Severe detoxification reactions with heart trouble, perspiration, trembling, tendency to cramps, restlessness, fear, despite beginning therapy gently. Immediate manual abdominal treatment results in furthering of elimination. Immediately afterwards, evacuation of bowels with relief, reactions diminish.

This increasingly cleanses all bodily juices and provides every cell of the body with more oxygen and high-quality nutrient solutions.

The manual abdominal treatment is also a breathing therapy. If there is a disorder in the digestive system, it must also be assumed that there is a disorder in breathing function. If the abdomen, especially an inflamed small intestine, obstructs the falling of the diaphragm during inhalation, breathing becomes more shallow, resulting in poor ventilation and airing of the lungs. Synchronizing the abdominal treatment with the patient's breathing utilizes natural changes in pressure between the chest and the abdomen as a driving force for intestinal activity, lymph circulation, and blood flow. Breathing therapy can bring decisive relief, especially for asthmatics.

Manual abdominal treatment is such an effective therapy encompassing the entire body that it should be carried out exclusively by a specially trained Mayr doctor.

The manual abdominal treatment is also a diagnostic check-up. The Mayr doctor, while treating the patient, always feels and examines sections of the digestive system to locate any burdened sections. Spasms, intestinal loops filled with faeces or gas, enlargement or congestion of the liver—everything is addressed during therapy. The Mayr doctor also checks whether changes meet expectations, and can recognize and assess detoxification reactions.

Supplementation

Today, we are exposed to a range of pressures from a variety of areas. The body's reaction to stress is fairly uniform, regardless of how different the causes of stress may be.

It is important to begin supplementation during Mayr therapy.

During its initial response to stress, the body tries to re-establish balance by mobilizing minerals, trace elements, and vitamins, because many regulatory processes require these substances. Normally, they are present in sufficient quantities and there are usually some reserves stored in the body. However, if stress continues for a longer period of time, or even increases—as is generally the case today—these minerals, trace elements, and vitamins are used up. The amount present in the body is reduced.

Another influencing factor is that our present-day nutritional habits do not supply our body with enough of these substances. Initial borderline deficiencies are hardly noticed by the person affected, and pronounced deficiencies are frequently misinterpreted. On the other hand, we require these minerals, trace elements, and vitamins, particularly in the case of allergies and intolerances, for gaining at least some control of the disorder. For example, we have already recognized that calcium, copper, vitamin C, and vitamin B6 are essential in the case of histamine intolerance. We have to assume that many people have deficiencies in these areas nowadays. Such deficiencies cannot be removed with even the most well implemented Mayr therapy. On the contrary, Mayr therapy itself, with its detoxification of the liver and neutralization of acids, requires these important substances. It is therefore important to begin supplementation during Mayr therapy.

To a minimal degree, Mayr himself had already begun to subconsciously pursue supplementation by making his patients drink Carlsbad water. Carlsbad water contains primarily sodium bicarbonate, as well as Glauber's salt and Epsom salts. Sodium bicarbonate is one of the most important substances for de-acidification. It is normally produced in the stomach, then passed on to the blood, and regulates the acid–base balance. Administering sodium bicarbonate is one of the most important therapeutic measures for treatment of allergies.

Orthomolecular Medicine

Preventing and treating disease by providing the body with optimal amounts of substances which are natural to the body is called orthomolecular medicine. The term "ortho" comes from the Greek language and means "correct, good"; molecules are the smallest functional particles in the body. Orthomolecular therapy provides the body with the right molecules in the right concentration. It encompasses the administering of minerals, trace elements, vitamins, fatty acids, amino acids, enzymes, and hormones. The term "orthomolecular" was coined by the two-time Nobel prize winner, Linus Pauling, who defined orthomolecular medicine as follows:

Definition	Orthomolecular medicine is the maintenance of good health and the treatment of illnesses by changing the concentration of substances present in the body.

Orthomolecular medicine, like modern Mayr medicine, is concerned with maintaining health as well as with treating illnesses.

Orthomolecular medicine works with high doses of supplements and should therefore be administered only under supervision of a doctor.

The principles of orthomolecular therapy have a long tradition in the treatment of illnesses. For example, anaemia due to iron deficiency is, of course, treated by administering iron. Diabetes is a deficiency of insulin, the enzyme responsible for the breakdown of sugar. Insulin can be supplemented with ortho-molecular therapy.

Somewhat more problematic is the use of orthomolecular therapy in the area of disease prevention. Although there is agreement as to the significance of various orthomolecular substances, such as vitamins and trace elements, it is widely assumed that "normal" nutrition assures an adequate supply of these substances. However, knowledge of the cardinal errors according to Mayr refutes this. The individual misdigestion processes alone use up such large quantities of orthomolecular substances in the digestive tract that only a minimal amount of the consumed quantity is actually absorbed.

I am asked daily about the necessity of taking orthomolecular substances. Do we have to take nutritional supplements, or are they adequately supplied by the food we eat?

The following is an example:
Details regarding the substances contained in individual foods can be found in various tables of nutritional values. These tables were compiled for the first time about 30–40 years ago, when interest in these substances first developed. Today, however, far fewer minerals are found in our food than several decades ago, due to changes in cultivation and fertilization methods, and exhaustion of arable soil. This has been confirmed in more recent investigations: Our foods today contain only about half the amount of substances given in the old tables. In addition, minerals and vitamins are lost to various degrees through the preparation and preservation of food.

Since our requirements have increased while our supply has not kept pace, appropriate individual supplementation is more important today than ever before.

Compounding this situation is that the quantities of these substances contained in foods are no longer the same as they were only one or two generations ago. Unbalanced agriculture, monoculture, fertilization, failure to keep animals in a manner that meets their needs, and pesticides have all contributed to this situation.

The question of requirement is also a question of drawing limits. Let us take vitamin C as an example: the U.S. Food and Nutrition Board of the National Academy of Sciences in 2000 set the recommended daily amounts of vitamin C at 90 milligrams per day for men and 75 mg a day for women. Before that, the "RDA" (recommended daily amount) was 60 mg a day. The European Community RDA is 60 mg. Similar levels are recommended in Australia. The Dietetic Societies of Germany, Austria, and Switzerland recommend a daily intake of 75 mg of vitamin C (recently they have begun to work up to 120 mg). These levels are expected to prevent the outbreak of scurvy (a disease dreaded by seafarers when they had no access to fresh vegetables for a longer period of time; it was prevented by sauerkraut, which is rich in vitamin C). On the one hand, one can assume this to be correct, because scurvy rarely occurs in Europe or North America. On the other hand, it is not an "ideal solution." Both in Mayr's way of thinking and in orthomolecular medicine, we base our assumptions on ideal relationships, which require higher levels of supplementation. Orthomolecular therapy frequently uses considerably higher doses for therapeutic purposes. For example, several grams are vitamin C per day are given to treat an infection or to lower histamine levels in cases of histamine intolerance.

Orthomolecular therapy needs to be conducted by a doctor experienced in this field. The administering of individual orthomolecular substances is explained in more detail in the discussion on allergy treatments.

Practical Application of Mayr Therapy for Treating Allergies/Intolerances

The key to practical implementation of Mayr therapy is the consideration of individual requirements. Mayr diagnostics, complemented by AK, enable the assessment of the patient's current state of health. The therapy modalities of rest and simplification, cleansing, training, and supplementation are always tailored strictly to the needs of the individual.

For a long time, Mayr therapy was equated with the "milk and bread roll cure." This cliché was never really applicable and must be completely thrown overboard today. The overriding principle of Mayr therapy is individualized dietetic recuperation. All possibilities are open here, from strict fasting all the way to the Mild Clearing Diet. Personal preferences and biochemical necessities are to be taken into consideration. For allergy treatment, this signifies the following:

Addressing Individual Needs

If a person does not like individual foods, for whatever reason, these are to be avoided during Mayr therapy. Participating in Mayr therapy is based on personal choice. If a Mayr doctor requires a patient to eat a certain food, no success will be achieved. In addition, the rejection of a food often indicates a food intolerance.

A craving for certain foods can indicate an addiction allergy.

With children, this connection is still very obvious. However, the opposite is also possible, where a craving exists for a food that is not tolerated. This is referred to as addiction allergy.

Rest and simplification can be accomplished by eating less food, but eating it correctly. Resting also means providing the body with the right foods, namely those that can be digested well. This naturally rules out untested or nontolerated foods. Conducting a Mayr therapy using foods that trigger an allergy is not in accordance with the principles of rest and simplification, but rather signifies maximum chemical stress. Therefore, tolerance of the foods used during therapy is tested using AK and the diet is adjusted accordingly.

With all therapeutic measures, it should be ensured that individual therapy components do not intensify, trigger, or prevent allergies from receding. Therefore, ideally, all measures such as foods, medication, herbs used for tea, orthomolecular substances, inhalants, skin ointments, bath additives etc., are tested to this effect by means of AK. Mayr therapy also signifies learning healthy eating habits again. Mayr himself described this in the quote below.

Quoting *F.X. Mayr*	...In order to give the human digestive system a rest, we use the digestive system of the cow as our diet kitchen...Milk contains everything that the animal and human body needs to grow and develop properly...However, it is important that the milk is not drunk but is sipped, small portions being put into the mouth with a teaspoon and properly mixed with saliva there. To encourage people who bolt their food to insalivate the milk well,...I ask them to them eat one or two bread rolls, as they wish, at every meal – three or four days old and air-dried. And I recommend cutting the bread rolls into small pieces and rolling each piece around in the mouth and chewing it up until it becomes a very thin pulp. This is then mixed with a small sip, a teaspoon full, of milk. The milk is then sucked out and swallowed; the pulp is chewed further and again mixed with milk etc. ...

Basic Principles of F.X. Mayr Therapy

- Milk is regarded as a food. Due to the substances contained in milk, a minimal amount supplies high-quality nutrients. Milk as a food today, however, is more problematic than in Mayr's days.
- As a liquid food, milk cannot be insalivated/digested properly. This is where the stale bread roll acts as a trainer for chewing, to prevent the milk from being gulped down.
- This points to the necessity of ensuring, during Mayr therapy, that a high-quality food like milk can be optimally digested.

With allergies, it will be necessary to find alternatives to milk and bread rolls that fulfil all therapeutic principles. Conventional bread and rolls are produced from wheat flour. Unfortunately, many bakers use ready-made baking mixes, the contents of which are not exactly known. Some individuals can react to these. However, it is easy to make bread from other cereal grains such as such as spelt, rye, oats, kamut, amaranth, or similar grain, in order to avoid wheat.

Bread rolls and many breads also contain yeast. In the case of a dysbiosis in the form of candidiasis, reactions to yeast are frequent. When yeast is omitted in the production of bread, the dough does not rise, resulting in round, flat bread loaves. These can also be made from spelt, rye, kamut, or other cereal grains.

If none of the cereal grains suitable for bread-baking are tolerated or in case of gluten intolerance (celiac disease), millet, maize, amaranth, or buckwheat is used.

250 g	finely-ground flour, freshly ground if possible, and sifted to remove any bran particles	*Basic Recipe for Flat Bread Loaves without Yeast*
0.5 l	carbonated mineral water sea salt, finely ground caraway or anise seeds	*(makes about 4 servings/loaves)*

Gently stir flour and mineral water together into a soft dough, then season. Spoon dough onto baking parchment to form four flat, round or oval loaves, using two wet spoons. Smooth loaves with a wet spoon. Pierce dough several times with a fork. Bake in a preheated oven at 220–250 C (400 to 450 degrees) for about 15 minutes, until loaves turn a nice color. Cool on a wire wrack, covered with a clean tea-towel, and allow to dry through (takes from several hours to a day, depending on climate).

Flat bread loaves should be eaten the same day, or they can be frozen and then removed from freezer about 30 minutes before they are needed.

These flat breads can be made from practically any kind of cereal grains, such as spelt, kamut, rye, buckwheat, maize, amaranth, and quinoa. Substituting mineral water with sheep's milk or acidophilus milk—provided they are suitably tolerated—is possible but not absolutely necessary. Flat breads can also be made using natural sour dough, but this requires a lot more effort.

Various kinds of crispbreads made with wheat alternatives, including ready-made amaranth crispbreads, are now available in bakeries, health food stores and even selected supermarkets, and offer a possible alternative.

Should it be necessary to avoid all kinds of cereal grains, as initially in the case of candidiasis, we can fall back on the potato. Here, a boiled potato is cut into slices and chewed thoroughly. Potatoes may, however, may be contraindicated in cases of intolerance to nightshade plants.

A similar procedure is necessary in the choice of other foods used during Mayr therapy. Mayr referred to milk as a high-quality food, which was absolutely correct in his day, but today's milk can no longer be rated in the same way. There are many reasons for this which would be beyond the scope of our considerations.

Important Considerations:
- Cow's milk constitutes one of the most frequent primary food allergens.
- Intolerances often occur in the course of a dysbiosis.
- Cow's milk protein is extremely indigestible for babies and therefore, tends not to be tolerated.
- Incomplete breakdown of cow's milk protein results in enteropathy and intestinal autointoxification.
- Cow's milk protein is changed through preservation such as pasteurization.
- Reactions in the form of lactose intolerance are possible.

All this leads to the conclusion that cow's milk, before being administered as a dietetic substance during a Mayr therapy, must be unconditionally tested for tolerance.

Alternatives to Cow's Milk:
- Sheep's milk, goat's milk, mare's milk
- Oat, rice, or soy milk
- Vegetable soup/base soup
- Various spreads such as vitamin spread, chestnut spread

We have now established that Mayr therapy can be carried out in varying degrees of intensity as indicated by Mayr diagnostics. We will now turn our attention to the most intensive form of Mayr therapy.

Water/Tea Fasting

Water/tea fasting is both possible and very effective under close medical supervision within the framework of in-patient Mayr therapy. All herbal teas selected need to be tested to assure they are well tolerated. Some plants, such as the nettle, have high levels of histamine and must therefore be avoided.

When making clear vegetable broth, it is important that only vegetables and ingredients that are well tolerated are used. The carrot is the most significant vegetable to be aware of (for cross-allergies with various pollen allergies, see p. 21). Potatoes can be involved in intolerance to night shade plants.

When taking tea or broth as a meal, it is recommended that both be spooned into the mouth, chewed and insalivated. This is not intended as harassment, but for training healthy chewing habits from the beginning of therapy.

Milk/Bread Roll Diet

This form of therapy has made Mayr therapy widely known. Mayr always intended it to include the training in chewing as an important therapeutic measure. With allergies, we have to keep to the fundamental principles of this diet, while adjusting the foods into address individual tolerances. This can be achieved by means of the AK test. The following are available as an alternative to the classic form:

Wheat roll	Spelt roll
	Rye crispbread
	Spelt flat breads
	Millet/amaranth flat breads
	Rice waffles
	Cornflakes (unsweetened)
	Potatoes

Cow's milk	Sour milk, yogurt
	Sheep's milk, sheep's milk yogurt, sheep's milk curd cheese
	Goat milk, goat milk yogurt
	Oat, rice, soy milk
	Base soup

It is important that these foods are taken in exactly the way that Mayr described. A small bite is taken of, for example, spelt flat bread, and this is chewed intensively and thoroughly until a liquid pulp of food and saliva is produced. Then small teaspoons of, for example, yogurt from sheep's milk is taken into the mouth, chewed further, mixed thoroughly, and swallowed. This procedure is repeated until a pleasant feeling of satiation occurs. Intervals of at least four to five hours must be observed between meals in order to give the body adequate opportunity to completely digest what has been eaten. Should feelings of hunger occur shortly before the next meal, this is to be viewed as a first indication of returning rhythms.

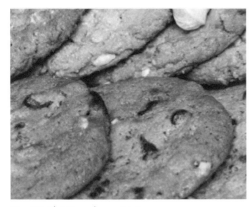
Fig. 17 Flat Breads are tasty.

As we know, digestive performance diminishes towards evening; therefore only a little herbal tea is spooned in the evening. A little honey can be dissolved in the tea, a slice of orange or lemon can also be added. But if we consider that honey, as a concentrated carbohydrate, has a tendency to ferment, it should be avoided by sensitive people with flatulence. In this case, a small piece of a spelt flat bread is often more beneficial than the concentrated honey.

We have been introduced to simplification as an important part of the Mayr therapy, meaning that the same food is always eaten. Although this also applies in the case of allergies, it has to be modified in some cases in favor of a rotation of foods. This is due to the malfunctioning of the immune system. It may react to the repeated exposure to one food by developing an intolerance to a previously well-tolerated food. In the case of a dysbiosis in the form of candidiasis, this rotation of foods (and medications) is absolutely necessary to achieve effectiveness.

During treatment, it will become apparent, for example through the manual abdominal treatment carried out by the doctor, if the expected improvement in abdominal results does not take place. Increased flatulence, spastic sections of the intestines, liver congestion, and signs of reintoxification are such indications. In the AK test, which is then carried out, the causes of changed muscle reactions can be found.

In the course of Mayr therapy, the patient is gradually given more to eat. This leads to the extended form of the milk/bread roll diet.

Extended Milk/Bread Roll Diet

Meals now become somewhat more sophisticated, while continuing to observe training in chewing and the therapy principles for acquiring healthy eating habits. The following are suitable as additional fare – again provided they are tolerated:

- Various spreads made from carrots and celery, curd cheese from sheep's milk
- Turkey breast, ham from beef, avocado (spread)
- Soft-boiled egg (possibly quail egg)
- Root vegetables
- Cold-pressed vegetable oils

Cold-pressed vegetable oils are especially important for many allergies. Not because of the calories they supply, but because of their many beneficial effects on the metabolism. These cold-pressed vegetable oils

- prevent inflammation (above all, linseed oil, hemp oil)
- act as a preliminary stage for the hormones of the adrenal glands (cortisone, progesterone)

- Activate the thymus gland as an organ of the immune system
- Sooth skin conditions such as neurodermatitis

Administering them as a supplement can lead to a decisive improvement in general condition, as well as reduce allergy symptoms.

Mild Clearing Diet

The Mild Clearing Diet is the ideal transition from intensive Mayr therapy to everyday fare. It is in keeping with the guidelines of rest and simplification, both in the choice and preparation of foods. Of course, it is no longer as intensive and monotony is also relaxed, but in comparison to the "jumble of everyday fare", the Mild Clearing Diet provides order in the daily menu.

The Mild Clearing Diet is also the ideal form of Mayr therapy for many people, when a more intensive diet is not possible. Because of its gently detoxification effect, it can be carried out over a longer period of time, which is of special advantage in the case of allergies. It is suitable for out-patient therapy and for the modification of nutritional habits at home. (Contact the Golf Hotel Health Center at the address at the end of this book for more information about the Mild Clearing Diet).

Important Considerations for Treating Allergies
- Fostering healthy eating habits; emphasis should be placed on the interplay between hunger and satiation.
- Breakfast corresponds approximately to the "extended milk/bread roll diet."
- Easily digestible meals are prepared at midday, for example potatoes and vegetables, fish and vegetables.
- Still as little as possible in the evening; at most some base soup or one of the supplemental items from the extended milk bread roll diet with bread.

It is important that only foods are eaten that have been shown to be tolerated.

Epsom Salts, Glauber's Salt
As previously explained, a glass of Epsom salts dissolved in warm water is drunk in the morning to cleanse the intestines and to further detoxify. In the case allergies or intolerance, it is not only theoretically conceivable but indeed not unusual that an intolerance to Epsom salts or Glauber's salt also occurs. It is therefore recommended that Epsom salts and Glauber's salt are also tested for tolerance by means of an AK test. Should this situation arise, intestinal cleansing must be carried out by other means, for example, by administering magnesium citrate, vitamin C, or bitter substances.

There is also a range of intolerances with herbal teas. The nettle has already been mentioned as a plant rich in histamine. In addition, however, reactions to individual plants frequently occur, which means that herbal teas are recommended to be tested by means of AK.

Chronological Sequence of Mayr Therapy for Allergies

For Mayr therapy to be meaningful requires at least 3 to 4 weeks. It will not be possible to improve the digestive system sufficiently for individual food intolerances to disappear within a shorter period of time. It has also proven advisable to plan on about 4 to 6 weeks of therapy for the treatment of dysbiosis in the form of candidiasis.

The treatment of parasite infestation can sometimes take even longer because the respective generation cycles must be taken into consideration. This does not mean 4 to 6 weeks of only the most intensive Mayr therapy. For example, the following course of treatment is both sensible and possible in practice:
- 1 week Mild Clearing Diet as a lead-in
- 2 weeks intensive diet in the form of milk/bread roll diet
- 1 to 2 weeks Mild Clearing Diet as transition

Or, on an in-patient basis:

- 3 weeks intensive milk/bread roll diet
- 1 to 2 weeks Mild Clearing Diet as transition

Chronological sequence—how long individual forms of diet are recommended and how the transition to everyday fare should take place—is very individual, as is Mayr therapy in general.

The question often arises as to when individual foods that are not tolerated can be eaten again. Any answers to this question are pure speculation. From experience, it can be said that it will take at least 4 to 6 weeks, and usually longer. Although the symptoms will have diminished or will no longer be present after this time, they would return immediately on consumption of the nontolerated food. Not until the condition of the digestive system has been improved to such an extent that it can again completely carry out its natural functions will it be possible for a previously nontolerated food to be eaten. This could well take 3, 6, or 12 months, or even longer.

Supportive Measures

We will find deficiencies of minerals, trace elements, and/or vitamins with many, if not all forms of allergy and intolerance. However, a definite improvement in symptoms will be noticed by administering the correct orthomolecular substance.

The following is again important for practical implementation of therapy:

Supplements in powder form without additives or capsules that can be opened and their contents poured out, are preferable to tablets or film tablets with coatings.

AK testing of all therapeutically relevant medication is necessary to test the individual rate of tolerance. Although a particular substance (e. g., zinc) may be absolutely necessary in many cases, its pharmaceutical preparation may contain fillers, binders, and various additives. The immune system can react to these additives, resulting not in a reduction but an increase in allergy symptoms. Therefore, as doctors, we must accustom ourselves to testing pure orthomolecular substances and subsequently using only these. This is the only way we can succeed in alleviating symptoms.

The following orthomolecular substances are important in the case of allergies:

Zinc

Zinc is found as a central mineral in many enzyme systems and influences the effect of the thymus gland as an immuno-competent organ. Zinc influences acid–base balance, supports hormone production of the adrenal glands (cortisone, progesterone) and is important in all skin disorders, including its attributes (hair, nails). Zinc is used with candidiasis/parasitosis, neutralizes heavy metals, and is almost always absent in cases of fructose intolerance.

Daily requirements: approximately 15 mg.

Therapeutic dosage: approximately 30–60 mg.

Calcium

Calcium is one of the most important mineral substances in cases of allergies. It reduces the effect of histamine. In addition, calcium is a component of bones and teeth, where it is responsible for strength and firmness (osteoporosis, periodontitis). Calcium is involved in the transfer of information to the cell walls; there is an increased tendency to cramp with calcium deficiency (tetany).

Daily requirements: approximately 1 g.

Therapeutic dose: approximately 1 g.

- **Important:** one cup of ground coffee eliminates about 6 mg of calcium!

Copper

Copper is stored in the liver and is one of our most important anti-inflammatory minerals. It is important in cases of histamine intolerance because breakdown of histamine is carried out through an enzyme containing copper (diamine oxidase or DAO). Copper deficiency or the increased requirement of copper due to inflammation intensify allergy symptoms.

Daily requirements: approximately 2 mg.
Therapeutic dosage: approximately 4–8 mg.
Copper is not to be taken simultaneously with zinc!

Sodium Bicarbonate

Sodium bicarbonate is the most important substance with inflammation. All inflammation involves local excess acidity. Sodium bicarbonate balances acidity, reduces excess acidity in the stomach, reduces pain, and has anti-inflammatory properties in cases of allergies. Taking sodium bicarbonate as a base powder between meals has proven to be worthwhile

- **Important:** with acute symptoms, sodium bicarbonate can be administered by intravenous infusion, which can quickly control symptoms. The best method of intake is as a base powder dissolved in water and drunk between meals.

Recipe for Base Powder		
	Sodium Monophosphate	10
	Potassium Citrate	10
	Calcium Carbonate	100
	Sodium Bicarbonate	200
	Therapeutic dose: 2–20 g per day.	

Vitamin B6

Vitamin B6 is important for the nerves and for the breakdown of protein. A diet rich in protein, as is usually found in the Western world, frequently leads to B6 deficiency. B6 acts as a co-factor in the breakdown of histamine.
Therapeutic dosage: approximately 50 mg per day as activated B6.

Vitamin C

Vitamin C is well known as being very effective with colds, minor infections, or viral inflammation. These all involve the immune system. With allergies, vitamin C lowers histamine levels, with quantities of about 2–10 g or more required to achieve this result. It is administered partially as an intravenous infusion, since when supplied via the digestive system, high doses result in soft stool or even diarrhea. The correct therapeutic dosage falls just short of causing diarrhea. It is arrived at by taking increasing amounts until diarrhea occurs, then slightly reducing the amount.

- **Important:** Vitamin C should be taken in buffered, pH-neutral form to avoid local acidic effects, and as a powder dissolved in water, possibly mixed with base powder. To buffer pure vitamin C, it can be mixed with base powder at a 1:1 ratio.

Vitamin F

Vitamin F means unsaturated fatty acids. These are of particular significance, especially in the case of allergies. They are important in all skin disorders, above all neurodermatitis, allergy eczema (contact eczema), and dry skin. Highly unsaturated fatty acids are preliminary stages for synthesis of the hormones cortisone and progesterone in the adrenal glands. The thymus gland depends on unsaturated fatty acids to provide information to specialized immuno cells. Fatty acids also have many metabolic functions without which healthy life is not possible.

Daily requirement: about 5–10 g (2 tablespoons) of cold-pressed vegetable oil.

- **Important**: highly unsaturated fatty acids require vitamin E as protection to prevent rancidity. Therefore intake of 200–400 IU of vitamin E is necessary daily. Light, air and heat destroy highly unsaturated fatty acids; therefore cold-pressed vegetable oil should be stored in dark bottles, well-sealed, in the refrigerator. Do not heat! If added to cooked foods, add just before serving.

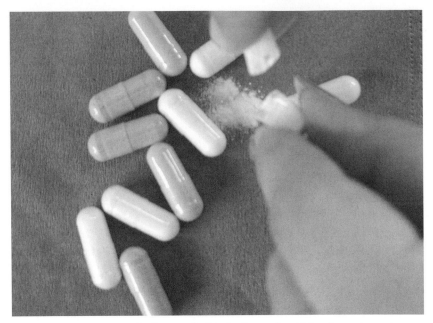

Fig. 18 All vitamins can also be supplied in the form of nutritional supplements.

Practical Tips for Allergy Treatment

Pollinosis, Neurodermatitis, Bronchial Asthma

This complex of illnesses is closely connected. Even new-born babies frequently have signs of cradle cap or develop mild skin symptoms during the first months of their lives. The mother's nutrition is a decisive factor as long as the child is breast fed. If the mother eats flatulence-causing food, the baby will also have flatulence. If the mother suffers from a food intolerance or allergy, there is a danger that, should she consume the nontolerated food, it will also have an effect on the baby via the mother's milk. An allergy or intolerance to cow's milk is found particularly with neurodermatitis and bronchial asthma. This applies to all cow's milk products, including yogurt, curd-cheese, cheese, and butter. If one of the parents is known to have neurodermatitis or bronchial asthma, it is recommended that the new-born baby be given no cow's milk products at all during the first year of life. This recommendation also applies to the mother as long as she is breast feeding.

Cradle cap—neurodermatitis—constant colds—frequent tonsillitis up to removal of the tonsils—frequent bronchitis, hay fever—then asthma. As a teenager or adult, alternating skin complaints and asthma.

Typical Illness Progression

How Mayr Therapy Can Help

Chinese medicine teaches that all toxins that cannot be eliminated via the intestines and kidneys are eliminated via the lungs and skin. Experience also shows that skin disorders, if suppressed, lead to disorders of the inner organs. In Mayr therapy, we will therefore attempt to relieve the lungs and the skin. This is done by stimulating elimination via the intestines and kidneys.

117

Epsom Salts, Colon Hydrotherapy, and Teas

Elimination via the intestines can be encouraged, not only with Epsom salts, but also with enemas or colon-hydrotherapy. In addition, bitter substances, vitamin C, and magnesium citrate are possible, higher doses of which can have a laxative effect.

Above all, plentiful intake of liquids is important for the kidneys. "Kidney teas" can provide additional support (solidago, berberis). Stimulation of kidney activity can also be achieved with foot reflex-zone treatment or the friction sit-bath according to Kuhne. (see p. 112)

Oils

Neurodermatitis involves an enzyme defect in the conversion of unsaturated fatty acids in about 50% of all cases. This underlines the significance of unsaturated fatty acids for therapy. Above all, the so-called dihomogamma-linolenic acid (DGLA), contained in borage oil or primrose oil, has good therapeutic effects. Black caraway seed oil (also known as black seed oil or nigella sativa), which also gently supports the thymus gland as the immune organ, can be very helpful. Therapeutic choice of the individual oils is made by means of the AK test.

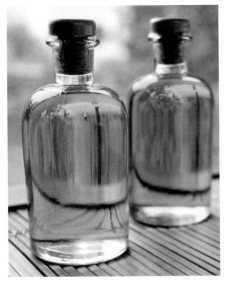

Fig. 19 Oils are great for skin care.

Local applications of cold-pressed vegetable oils are important with all skin disorders, including those of nonspecific eczema. Oils can be used to moisturize the skin, as a bath supplement, or as oil compresses. In most cases, the use of oil is more pleasant than that of skin creams, and more importantly, oils do not impede elimination through the skin. Many creams clog skin pores and thus prevent effective detoxification.

Only fresh, cold-pressed vegetable oils that have been tested for tolerance should be used; old oils not only smell unpleasantly rancid, but are also therapeutically unsuitable. They burden the metabolic process more than being therapeutically useful.

Addition of cold-pressed oils to meals is essential with all skin disorders. This is easily done in Mayr therapy by adding oil to base soups, or as a supplement in the Mild Clearing Diet.

Unsaturated fatty acids seek light and oxygen. In the metabolic process, they therefore wander as far as the skin, where they are then oxidized. Not until this happens does the skin gain proper smoothness. The intake of vitamin E, as a supplement to the oils, is important for oxidation protection.

Base Baths
help the skin to eliminate acids. About one handful of sodium bicarbonate (e. g., baking soda) is added to the bath water. Remain in the water for about 20 to 30 minutes, while water temperature is gradually increased. (Be careful of blood circulation—not too hot during Mayr therapy!) The appropriate addition of oils (tested for tolerance!) has a moisturizing effect on the skin. In the case of pronounced skin disorders, baths must be handled with extreme care, and it is absolutely essential to first stimulate detoxification via the intestines.

Inhalations, Nasal Reflex Therapy
support the lungs. Nasal reflex therapy was originated by Dr. Nils Krack. This therapy involves treating the mucous membranes of the nose with essential oils, which cleanses not only the nose region, but also the sinuses and the entire breathing tract. The oils used should be tested for tolerance by means of AK.

Food Test for Cases of Pollinosis
In the case of hay fever, or pollinosis, a food test is always necessary because of the many possibilities of cross-allergies between pollen and various foods. In most cases, a distinct improvement or complete disappearance of symptoms is achieved when the nontolerated foods are omitted for a sufficient period of time.

Heart–Circulatory Complaints

Of course, not all heart complaints can be explained by an allergy. However, we have seen that one of the effects of histamine is directed at the heart–circulatory system. Often, a person with heart problems knows that cardiac arrhythmia can occur following the consumption of nontolerated foods. In Mayr therapy, palpitations after meals should give cause to consider allergies. In this context, the work of the cardiologist Coca is interesting. Coca defined a food as being not tolerated when, following consumption of the food, the heartbeat increases by ten beats. Everyone can easily test this. The following self-check, after brief practice, is a good method for recognizing food intolerance.

Coca Test	Take your pulse before and again about 20 to 30 minutes after the meal (e. g. on your wrist or neck). If the pulse increases by more than 10 beats after the meal, you have not tolerated part of the meal

Histamine, in high doses, also lowers blood pressure. Constant tiredness is a frequent indication of food intolerance, because blood pressure does not really gain momentum. This effect can be observed in many places such as such as lectures, events, seminars, or simply in the office: following a meal, many people are extremely drowsy. The reason for this drowsiness is not because the blood sinks to the abdomen during digestion, but because of histamine that has not been broken down. Although a subsequent cup of coffee provides the adrenal glands with an impetus to "kick in," it causes the histamine problem to worsen.

Mayr therapy can eliminate such regulatory disorders quickly and effectively, increase vitality, and end the unpleasant symptoms caused by food. Supplementation with calcium and, above all, potassium and magnesium as supportive measures in cases of cardiac arrhythmia are particularly important.

Patient A.P., female, age 58

Symptoms: heart complaints for the last 12 years, fluttering of the heart after every meal, hypertonia, tendency to constipation, tiredness.

Mayr Diagnostics: massive radix edema, spastic large intestine, blotchy tongue.
AK Test Results: generalized high blood pressure, histamine intolerance, weakness of the adrenal glands, positive reaction to calcium, copper, vitamin B6, and vitamin C. In addition, parasite infestation.
Food Test Results: intolerance to cow's milk products, wheat, fructose, and fish.

During Mayr Therapy: heart complaints as a reaction to detoxification. After 3 weeks of in-patient Mayr therapy, distinct improvement. No heart complaints at all after meals. After 4 months avoidance of the foods, only cow's milk is still not tolerated; no new heart problems.

Migraines, Headaches

Mayr therapy is very often carried out in cases of headaches or migraine. On the other hand, headaches are also a frequent if not regular detoxification symptom during Mayr therapy.

It has been shown that headaches occur in a direct relationship to histamine levels. In many cases, migraine or headache sufferers also make a link to individual foods.

When a migraine begins, the race against time also begins. If the circulating toxins (histamine, biogenic amines) can be successfully eliminated via the intestines, this reduces the symptoms. For this reason, enemas and/or colon hydrotherapy are also recommended. The friction sit-bath according to Kuhne also helps by stimulating elimination "downward."

Headaches always indicate excess local acidity. Base powders and zinc, in large quantities, produce good results. Both can be administered as intravenous infusion in case of acute and severe symptoms. Neural-

Friction ***Sit-Bath*** ***According to*** ***Kuhne***	The friction sit-bath promotes elimination via the uro-genital region. This is especially important with allergies for skin symptoms or intestinal complaints. The person bathing sits on a bucket of water or on the bidet. The water initially has a pleasant temperature. The genital region is rinsed or gently washed using a bath-sponge or simply a hand. This is done for at least 20 minutes daily, whereby the temperature of the water should be increasingly lowered, so that the person bathing tolerates cold water too, and finds it pleasant. Should the person not tolerate cold water, hot water can also be used.

therapeutic infiltration or acupuncture treatments can also be usefully applied during the detoxification phase. The liver, as an important detoxification agent, needs to be supported in every case. Base powders, various foods, and glutathione are helpful.

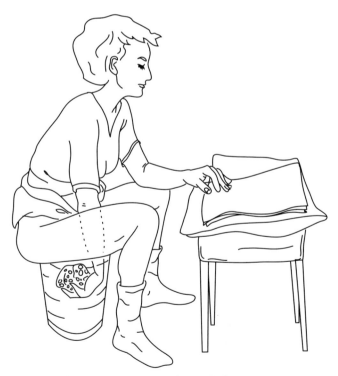

Fig. 20 Friction sit-bath for women according to Kuhne

If a tendency to develop migraines is already known from the case history, the above-mentioned measures should be carried out prophylactically at the beginning of Mayr therapy.

Disorders of the Digestive System

Almost all forms of digestive disorder are found with allergies and intolerances. Spastic colon, irritable bowels, both unspecific and specific inflammation, even disorders such as Crohn's disease and ulcerative colitis can be included. The one thing these all have in common is that they can be allergically induced.

In all cases, consistent implementation of Mayr therapy is useful to alleviate symptoms. Manual abdominal treatment by the doctor should be carried out daily wherever possible, and even twice daily in acute cases. Heat can be extremely helpful, but it can produce the opposite effect with some forms of inflammation. Individual requirements must be taken into consideration.

Frequent bowel movements indicate concentrated toxins in the rectum. Drinking plenty of clear liquids, base powder to neutralize acids and enemas are important relieving measures.

If cramps develop, calcium, magnesium, and copper have an outstanding effect—these are all orthomolecular substances indicated with histamine intolerance.

Candidiasis and parasites constitute a frequent burdening. Nevertheless, candidiasis develops a certain momentum of its own and, from a certain point on, demands specific treatment. It is important that candidiasis is considered in all cases of

> Candidiasis is always a consequence and never a primary cause.

suspicious intestinal symptoms. Strong essential oils of spices are helpful in treatment (cinnamon, garlic, cloves).

Parasites live in generation cycles. Regularly occurring symptoms, with intervals of very few symptoms, are a frequent indication of parasites, as is itching of the anus. Essential oils support the treatment of parasites, as do bitter substances such as Swedish bitters, black walnut tincture, yarrow, mugwort, and cloves.

Rheumatic Disorders, Arthritis

Rheumatism means simply "aching pain." This diagnosis is often used to describe disorder when the cause is unclear or not quite certain. Many "modern" diagnoses, such as polymyalgia syndrome or fibromyalgia, describe only where the pain is.

All rheumatic disorders have one thing in common: inflammation. It takes place in various tissues and causes pain. One possible cause of the inflammation is allergies. Experience shows that Mayr therapy brings a distinct improvement of symptoms in all cases. The prognosis with so-called "sero-negative arthritis or rheumatism" is very good, since it is frequently triggered by food intolerance or allergy. Of course, many rheumatic disorders are simply an overstraining of the connective tissue as a storage organ, and also respond very well to Mayr therapy.

A sufficient supply of bases is important to counteract the localized excess acidity. Base powder should be taken as often as possible; in cases of acute pain, it can also be administered as an intravenous infusion if necessary.

Detoxification is also promoted by base baths. Their benefit is twofold: warmth and immediate deacidification via the skin. Many are amazed at the rings of dirt left behind by the bath water even though appropriate hygienic measures were undertaken.

Of the minerals, copper must be mentioned above all. It is the most important anti-inflammatory mineral. Copper bracelets have been recommended from time to time in cases of joint disorders. Taking copper as

---

Patient A.M., female, age 48 | *Patient History*

Symptoms: musculoskeletal problems for about 2 years; last diagnosis: fibromyalgia. Treatment with a wide variety of different pain medications and immune suppressants. Recently, treatment for depression. Despite this, no improvement in pain. In laboratory tests, high IgE and eosinophilia.

Mayr Diagnostics: enlarged liver, severely inflamed small intestine, spastic large intestine. Overall congestion incl. liver, radix edema, edemas in lower legs.
AK *Test Results:* high blood pressure, histamine intolerance, parasites.
Food Test Results: intolerance to cow's milk products, rye, carrots, and walnuts. Weakness in entire hormonal system.

Mayr Therapy: Three weeks strict in-patient Mayr therapy, avoidance of nontolerated foods, orthomolecular supplementation. *After 1 week*: no pain in musculoskeletal system, patient can walk normally again, can go for walks. *After 3 weeks*: distinct improvement in abdominal results, continuation of orthomolecular supplementation. Support of adrenal glands. *Check-up after 3 months*: still no symptoms, good mobility, hormone system has recovered. Still histamine intolerance, intolerance to cow's milk, rye and carrots remains, no parasite infestation, normal immunoglobulin.

---

a nutritional supplement is far more effective. Copper is also necessary for the breakdown of histamine. In addition, zinc, calcium, magnesium, and fatty acids from cold-pressed vegetable oils, which also intervene directly in the inflammatory process, are important. The highly unsaturated fatty acids of the group of omega-3 oils—linseed oil, hemp oil, and fish oil—are, above all, natural suppliers of these fatty acids.

Those who do not like the taste of linseed oil can mix the oil with (sheep's) curd-cheese and almond paste. This is an outstanding mix, even during Mayr therapy but also later. Supplemented with fruit, it makes a wonderful breakfast.

Vitamin E also has anti-inflammatory effects. High doses (approximately 1200–1600 IU) can be administered initially. Its effects can be compared with those of common pain medication (aspirin). A maximum of 400 IU is beneficial in the long term.

Menstrual Disorders (Dysmenorrhea)

Women frequently complain of severe pain at the beginning of their menstrual period, which is not, or only inadequately, alleviated with common pain medications.

Histamine effects the smooth muscular system—mostly bronchial tubes (asthma) and intestines (irritable bowels)— but to some extent also the uterus. From a statistical point of view, consumption of eggs and cheese increase the risk of dysmenorrhea (painful menstrual periods). Jarisch was able to show that a reduction in the breakdown of histamine takes place immediately prior to the period. This can be a factor for the symptoms mentioned. In Mayr therapy, we frequently observe a normalization of menstruation, both in regularity and in symptoms. During Mayr therapy, menstruation can be premature or also delayed—depending on the need for detoxification.

Cramp-like disorders respond well to magnesium, copper, and vitamin B6—again, important orthomolecular substances in histamine intolerance. Many women also report that when they refrain from eating certain foods, their menstruation problems disappear.

Pregnancy

Pregnancy is an important consideration in the context of allergies. During pregnancy, the activity of the enzyme responsible for the breakdown of histamine (diamine oxidase or DOA) is multiplied severalfold. In addition, the adrenal gland of the child helps the mother to cope with allergy symptoms. These are reasons why allergies and intolerances are alleviated during pregnancy or may even appear have vanished.

Premature labor should give cause to consider a food intolerance. Everything that is not tolerated should be strictly avoided during pregnancy, to avoid problems for the growing child.

With knowledge of all these factors, Mayr therapy can be carried out without problem during pregnancy. In fact, man pregnancy disorders can even be avoided or treated with Mayr therapy.

Allergies and Sports Injuries

An allergy or intolerance leads to inflammation. This takes place in the connective tissue. Connective tissue is also the area of the muscles and tendons that are impacted in a wide variety of ways through exercise. Every inflammation constitutes a weak point that is not optimally resilient.

Exercise or athletics are frequently taken too far today, especially by recreational athletes who think they have to conduct themselves like world champions. This has turned exercise into a stress factor for many, one that can be a contributing factor for allergies.

In the section on AK, we saw that every muscle represents an inner organ (system) and vice-versa, for example the front thigh muscle (quadriceps) represents the small intestine and the hip abductor (tensor fasciae latae) of the thigh represents the large intestine. When we consider that allergies have a biochemical background in the digestive system, symptoms often become apparent on these skeletal thigh muscles.

Knee problems frequently occur with allergies because the base of the tendons constitute weak points. The overload caused by the allergy then leads to damage to the knee, meniscus, or musculoskeletal system.

Unfortunately, the nutrition of our much acclaimed athletes is not necessarily optimal. Overstraining in sports leads to excess acidity in the tissue and thus a tendency towards reduced resilience, pain, and danger

Patient History	**Patient E.H., female, age 34**

Symptoms: pain in left knee. Diagnosis by orthopedic surgeon: inflammatory state of irritation, damage to meniscus (knee cartilage) and cyst. Surgery to repair damage. Subsequent increase in pain, limited mobility, feeling of swelling. Secondary results: constipation.

Mayr Diagnostics: inflammation of small intestine, radix edema.
AK Test Results: generalized high blood pressure, histamine intolerance.
Food Test Results: wheat intolerance.

Mayr Therapy: Four weeks of Mild Clearing Diet, addressing wheat intolerance, calcium supplementation. After 1 week, swelling in knee has disappeared, pain decreases. After 4 weeks, no knee symptoms at all, all abdominal results improved. Patient very well, movement without pain, resumes exercise.

of injuries. Frequent cases of torn muscle fibers confirm this, and more so considering that the muscular system of the calf represents the adrenal gland. It is precisely this region that is the first to be overtaxed and injured in the case of exhaustion (weakness of the adrenal gland).

Athletes or physically active people use up more minerals, trace elements, and vitamins than other people because of their increased physical activity. They must therefore ensure an appropriately increased supply of these substances. Taking care of and advising athletes demands good understanding of the physiological and medical interrelations of sports medicine. It is, however, indisputable that sensible nutrition is just as much a prerequisite for the success of an athlete as specific training. Ignoring allergies results in a lowering of performance.

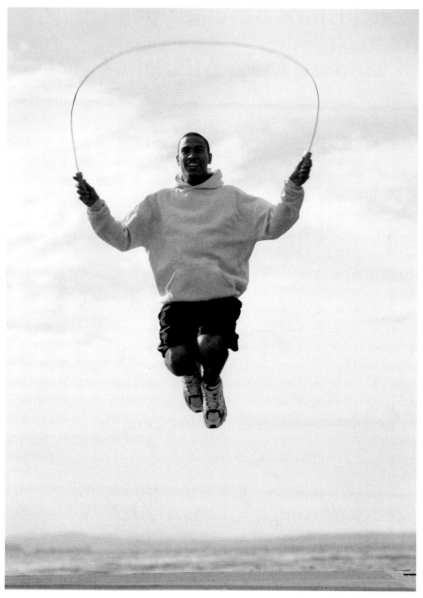

Fig. 21 Athletes and physically active people require a sensible diet.

Conclusions for Everyday Living from the Ideas of Modern Mayr Medicine

Mayr therapy is carried out for a certain length of time based on the findings of Mayr diagnostics, and in keeping with individual require- ments and necessity. As a medical therapy, Mayr therapy does not meet the criteria for healthy nutrition in everyday life. It would be completely wrong to conclude, for example, that the therapeutic use of milk and bread rolls constitutes a healthy form of everyday nutrition. Rather, Mayr therapy is designed to help regain healthy eating habits.

During and as a result of the Mayr therapy, we rediscover a great deal of sensitivity toward the workings of our own body. We recognize the exact point at which a pleasant feeling of satiation occurs, perceive healthy feelings of hunger before a meal, and learn to taste and enjoy food again. Allergy sufferers becomes much more intensely aware of which food is tolerated and which causes an allergic reaction, because they learn to recognize their special allergy symptoms. This sensitivity is an advantage and should not tempt us to say, "I don't tolerate anything at all now." Instead, we should tell ourselves, "I now react almost imme- diately and/or I react strongly." Recognizing and accepting this normal and important reaction is also an important experience in Mayr therapy.

Good Health through Living with Full Awareness following F.X. Mayr Therapy

The aim of Mayr therapy is healthier nutrition and a healthier lifestyle. Training is therefore the most important part of therapy. Healthy eating habits are intensively practiced during Mayr therapy, and old habits re- placed by new ones to promote lasting and consistent results for everyday living. This is of particular significance for those suffering from allergies. Allergies develop particularly often because of an enteropathy according to Mayr, with misdigestion in the form of fermentation or putrefaction, with subsequent intestinal autointoxification. The better the situation in the digestive system, the less likely is the tendency to develop an allergy. Every individual is responsible for nurturing healthy eating habits. Whether we chew well, insalivate our food, give ourselves time to digest properly, or "eat on the run" lies within the realm of personal responsibility with all its consequences. Allergy sufferers have to rethink their approach to food. If you are accustomed to attributing the blame for your allergy to food, you regain this responsibility during Mayr therapy, at least for the eating part of the process. Healthy nutrition is the combined result of food consumption and individual digestive performance.

Allergies or intolerances are decisively influenced by digestive performance. They frequently develop as a result of ignoring this rule. The good news is that allergies or intolerance can also be made to subside in the same way.

Mayr therapy is the beginning of a nutritional reorientation. The nontolerated foods are, of course, avoided in the case of allergies. It will take considerable time until all intestinal functions work optimally again. The following simple principles for everyday life arise as a consequence of Mayr therapy.

Avoiding All Raw Fruit and Vegetables in the Evening

We previously mentioned that digestive performance is at its lowest in the evening. It is therefore important to avoid anything that would over-tax our digestive performance in the evening. Raw fruit and vegetables demand a high degree of digestive performance because of they are a living food. If this digestive performance is not available at the time the food is eaten, misdigestion develops in the form of fermentation or putrefaction. Both of these have serious consequences for allergy sufferers: an increase in allergy symptoms.

We realize that various nutritional experts claim that people need plenty of vitamins. Although this recommendation is basically correct, evening is not the right time to meet this need. Therefore, in the evening consciously avoid salads, fresh fruit juices and desserts with fresh fruit. What should we eat in the evening? Mediterranean cuisine, for example, has much to offer:

- Steamed or grilled vegetables in olive oil as a starter (can be well-spiced)
- Fish or meat with vegetables
- Potato dishes
- ...anything, as long as it isn't raw foods!

Meat or fish with cooked vegetables is more easily digested in the evening than other foods. This is in accordance with the principles of food separation, where protein and carbohydrates are not eaten together in concentrated form at one meal. Food separation facilitates improved digestion.

Preparation of Easy-to-Digest Food
The art of healthy cuisine lies in preparing dishes in a way that preserves as many of the substances contained in foods as possible and makes them easily digestible. In addition, food should and must taste good, or nobody will accept changes in foods or preparation methods. The Mild Clearing Diet ideally meets all these requirements. (Contact the Golf Hotel Health Center at the address at the end of this book for more information about the Mild Clearing Diet).

With allergies, attention not only to the choice of food, but also to food preparation, is of special importance. Canned (tinned) or preserved foods, dishes using a combination of fat and flour (such as roux), as well as breaded and deep-fried foods are difficult to digest, very burdensome and always problematic. Instead, steamed, stir-fried, or simmered vegetables are considerably more suitable. Meat or fish can likewise be grilled, stir-fried or steamed. These cooking methods preserve the food's valuable ingredients and make them easily digestible. They also save calories while at the same time improving dishes like soups and sauces, all without overburdening the digestive system (see p. 89).

Choice of Foods

The following aspects should also be kept in mind:

Organic food and food derived from animals kept in a manner that meets their needs is of a much higher quality and preferable to food produced with conventional methods of agriculture and raising livestock. This has been confirmed in numerous tests and investigations. Wherever possible, organic foods should always be chosen.

Meat, fish, and cheese are concentrated protein-giving foods that should not be consumed in excessive quantities. In addition to their high protein content, protein-giving foods are also acid-producing. For this reason, it is recommended to combine them with base-producing foods. These include primarily vegetables, potherbs, ripe, locally grown fruit, and cold-pressed vegetable oils.

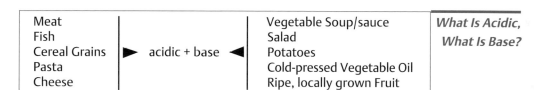

Meat			Vegetable Soup/sauce	*What Is Acidic,*
Fish			Salad	*What Is Base?*
Cereal Grains	▶ acidic + base ◀		Potatoes	
Pasta			Cold-pressed Vegetable Oil	
Cheese			Ripe, locally grown Fruit	

Allergies are pathological reactions to protein. Food freshness plays an important part. Foods that have been stored for a longer time, and certainly if stored for too long, should be avoided because of their possibly elevated histamine content.

High-quality, cold-pressed vegetable oils are essential for achieving long-term health improvements with allergies. Many of the toxins involved in allergies are fat-soluble. In addition, the barrier function of the intestines is also influenced by the quality of fat. Skin complaints require fats for therapy. Fats are therefore an indispensable part of comprehensive allergy treatment and prophylaxis.

Cold-pressed vegetable oils, although more expensive than conventional oils, are more substantial. Reducing the consumption of animal products will reduce the overall consumption of fat. Therefore, about two tablespoons of a good cold-pressed vegetable oil should be added to the diet daily.

It is best to purchase the oil in small, dark bottles. Good, cold-pressed extra virgin olive oil can also be bought in cans (tins). Look for terms like "cold-pressed," "first pressing," "unrefined," "natural, unadulterated," "unheated," "unfiltered," "naturally expeller-pressed" or "without toxic chemicals, solvents or preservatives." These terms need to be stated on the label, otherwise there is no guarantee that the bottle actually contains pure, unadulterated, cold-pressed oil. Make sure the oil is well-sealed and kept in the refrigerator, and that it is used as soon as possible after being opened. Light, air, and heat destroy these high-quality oils.

Cereal grains and the dishes made from them are important suppliers of mineral substances. Whole grain (wholemeal) products are better in the long-term than refined (white) flour products. This assumes that the grain is processed fresh and ground as finely as possible. Products containing whole, unmilled kernels of grain, for example bread with whole grain kernels or muesli or granola made with grain flakes or coarsely milled grain, are extremely difficult to digest. Only with a healthy digestive system and good digestive performance will it be possible to really digest these foods. In comparison, finely-ground, whole grain flour is easy to digest and is therefore recommended for everyday use. Millet, maize, quinoa, and amaranth are easily digestible and they are excellent for the preparation of a wide range of dishes. Grains, like protein foods, should be combined with vegetables to maintain acid–base balance.

The most important ingredient, however, remains healthy eating habits. This starts with setting a pleasing table and sitting down quietly to eat. Loving preparation of meals includes the way the food is presented on the plate: "The eyes also partake of the food." In an agreeable environment, it will be easier to enjoy meals through good chewing and insalivation, and to stop eating when the food tastes best and a pleasant feeling of satiation sets in.

Since we know that even the best intentions lose their effectiveness after a while, it is necessary to repeat the Mayr therapy from time to time. This is important for health in general, and essential in cases of allergy or intolerance. The therapy can be carried out regularly 1 day a week, and in addition, once a year for 3 or 4 weeks. With a "four year plan," even serious health disorders can be influenced positively.

Support of the metabolic process with orthomolecular substances needs to take place over a longer period of time. Interim check-ups—using Mayr diagnostics and AK—are necessary and a matter of course, because the need for individual substances frequently changes over time and supportive measures may need to be adjusted

Mayr Once Described the Effects of His Therapy in the Following Way:
"If you want to succeed in getting out of the valley of not feeling well and reach the mountain of health, I will point the way for you, will decide whether you are to take the steep ascent of strict fasting or the winding road of the milk/bread roll diet, or the Mild Clearing Diet, and will show you where to place your feet. I will always be by your side, be your friend, your mountain guide, but not your packhorse. You have to walk yourself!"

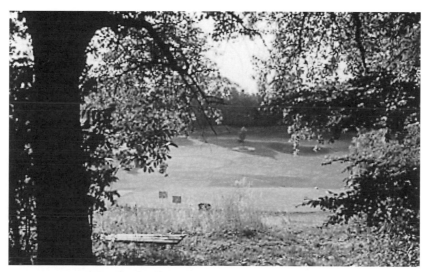

May this book accompany you on your way.

Appendix

About the Author

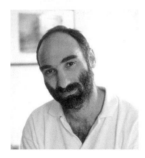

Dr. Harald Stossier entered the medical profession in a roundabout way. After graduating from a technical institute for electrical engineering, he worked as an electrical engineer for several years. During this time, he became aware that this work did not really provide him with fulfillment. So he followed his vocation and began to study medicine at the universities of Innsbruck and Graz.

During his studies, he became extensively involved in the methods of complimentary medicine. He undertook training in manual medicine, homeopathy, neural therapy, and applied kinesiology. He learned the methods of Mayr diagnostics and therapy under Dr. Erich Rauch, with whom he worked in the Golf Hotel Health Center in Dellach on Lake Wörth, Austria, since 1990. He took over from Dr. Rauch as Medical Director of the Health Center in 1996. Since then, Dr. Stossier has modernized Mayr therapy and adapted it to the special requirements of people suffering from allergies.

Today, Dr. Stossier is President of the International Society of Mayr Doctors and President of the International Medical Society for Applied Kinesiology. He is working for the establishment of both methods in the medical field.

Dr. Stossier is the consultant for complimentary medicine to the General Medical Council both of Carinthia and of Austria. He is also presently advisor for complementary medicine to the Austrian General Medical Council.

The author's address:
Dr. Harald Stossier
c/o Gesundheitszentrum Golfhotel am Wörthersee
A-9082 Maria Wörth-Dellach, Carinthia

Addresses

International Society of Mayr Doctors
Golfstraße 2
A-9082 Maria Wörth-Dellach
Austria

Tel: ++43 (0) 4273 2511–44
Fax: ++43 (0) 4273 2511–72
E-mail: office@fxmayr.com
Homepage: www.fxmayr.com

**IMAK—International Medical
Society for Applied Kinesiology**
Ärztekammer für Kärnten
(General Medical Council for
Carinthia)
St. Veiterstraße 34
A-9020 Klagenfurt
Austria

Tel: ++43 (0) 463 5856–35
Fax: ++43 (0) 463 514222
E-mail: office@imak.co.at
Homepage: www.imak.co.at

Golf Hotel Health Center
Golfstraße 2
A-9082 Maria Wörth-Dellach
Austria

Tel: ++43 (0) 4273 2511–43
Fax: ++43 (0) 4273 2511–72
E-mail: medizin@golfhotel.at
Homepage: www.golfhotel.at